IN 100 HEALTHY DISHES
we will star A Journey from
Snacks to Desserts

which will present 100 ideas for healthy meals across various categories, including Snacks, Salads, Soups, Main Courses, and more.

If you have allergies to certain ingredients, you can substitute them with suitable alternatives and adjust the ingredients according to your preferences

BY: E. Eshra

If you would like to get in touch, or have any questions or comments, then please send me an email at the following address:
pro.education.edu@gmail.com

© 2024 E. Eshra. ALL RIGHTS RESERVED.

No part of this book may be reproduced, distributed, or transmitted in any form or by any means, including photocopying, recording, or other electronic or mechanical methods, without the prior written permission of the publisher, except in the case of brief quotations embodied in critical reviews and certain other noncommercial uses permitted by copyright law.

Table of Contents

INTRODUCTION 4
- Introduction to the book

SNACKS 5
- Greek Yogurt with Honey and Berries
- Almonds and Dried Fruit Mix
- Apple Slices with Peanut Butter
- Veggie Sticks with Hummus
- Hard-Boiled Eggs
- Air-Popped Popcorn
- Cheese and Whole Grain Crackers
- Edamame
- Fruit Salad
- Dark Chocolate
- Cucumber Slices with Tzatziki
- Sweet Potato Chips
- Protein Bars
- Fruit and Nut Mix
- Rice Cakes with Avocado
- Baked Apple Chips
- Cottage Cheese with Pineapple
- Carrot and Celery Sticks
- Yogurt Parfait
- Frozen Grapes

SALADS 26
- Classic Caesar Salad
- Greek Salad
- Quinoa and Black Bean Salad
- Spinach and Strawberry Salad
- Kale and Avocado Salad
- Chickpea and Tomato Salad
- Mixed Greens with Balsamic Vinaigrette
- Roasted Beet Salad
- Asian Slaw
- Caprese Salad

WRAPS AND SANDWICHES 37
- Turkey and Avocado Wrap
- Chicken Caesar Wrap
- Veggie Hummus Wrap
- Tuna Salad Sandwich
- Caprese Sandwich
- Greek Pita Pocket
- Buffalo Chicken Wrap
- Egg Salad Sandwich
- Black Bean and Corn Wrap
- Turkey and Swiss Sandwich

SOUPS 48
- Tomato Basil Soup
- Lentil Soup
- Butternut Squash Soup
- Chicken and Vegetable Soup
- Minestrone Soup
- Spinach and White Bean Soup
- Broccoli Cheddar Soup
- Chicken Tortilla Soup
- Potato Leek Soup
- Roasted Red Pepper Soup
- Corn Chowder
- Gazpacho

MAIN MEALS 61
- Baked Salmon with Lemon
- Stuffed Bell Peppers
- Chicken Stir-Fry
- Sweet Potato and Black Bean Chili
- Grilled Chicken with Rice
- Spaghetti Squash with Marinara
- Shrimp Tacos
- Vegetable Curry
- Turkey Meatballs

- Vegetable Lasagna

- Grilled Veggie Skewers

- Lemon Herb Chicken

- Stuffed Zucchini Boats

- Air Fryer Chicken and Veggie Mix

- Baked Tilapia

- Vegetable Paella

- Turkey Stuffed Peppers

- Cauliflower Fried Rice

- BBQ Chicken

- Mushroom Risotto

Smoothies 82

- Berry Banana Smoothie

- Green Detox Smoothie

- Mango Pineapple Smoothie

- Strawberry Oat Smoothie

- Peanut Butter Banana Smoothie

- Avocado Spinach Smoothie

- Blueberry Almond Smoothie

- Tropical Kale Smoothie

- Chocolate Protein Smoothie

- Coconut Berry Smoothie

- Orange Carrot Smoothie

- Kiwi Spinach Smoothie

- Peach Ginger Smoothie

- Apple Cinnamon Smoothie

- Raspberry Chia Smoothie

- Pineapple Coconut Smoothie

- Cherry Vanilla Smoothie

- Pumpkin Spice Smoothie

- Lemon Blueberry Smoothie

- Banana Almond Smoothie

Desserts 103

- Chia Seed Pudding

- Fruit Sorbet

- Dark Chocolate Almond

- Apple Crisp

- Baked Pears with Honey

- Frozen Yogurt

- Chocolate Avocado Mousse

- Banana Oat Cookies

Conclusion 112

- Main points of the book

Introduction

Healthy eating doesn't have to be complicated or bland. By focusing on whole foods and balanced nutrition, you can enjoy a variety of delicious and satisfying meals that support your overall well-being. This e-book, "100 HEALTHY DISHES," offers 100 healthy meal ideas, each designed to provide essential nutrients while keeping calories in check. From snacks and smoothies to salads, wraps, and main courses, you'll find plenty of inspiration to make healthier choices every day. Whether you're looking to maintain your weight, boost your energy, or simply enjoy more wholesome meals, this collection has something for everyone.

If you find that you don't have all the necessary ingredients for a particular meal, don't worry. You can always look for other healthy alternatives to replace the unavailable ingredients. This flexibility allows you to adapt recipes to what you have on hand while still maintaining their nutritional value and deliciousness.

Let's dive in and discover the joy of healthy eating together.

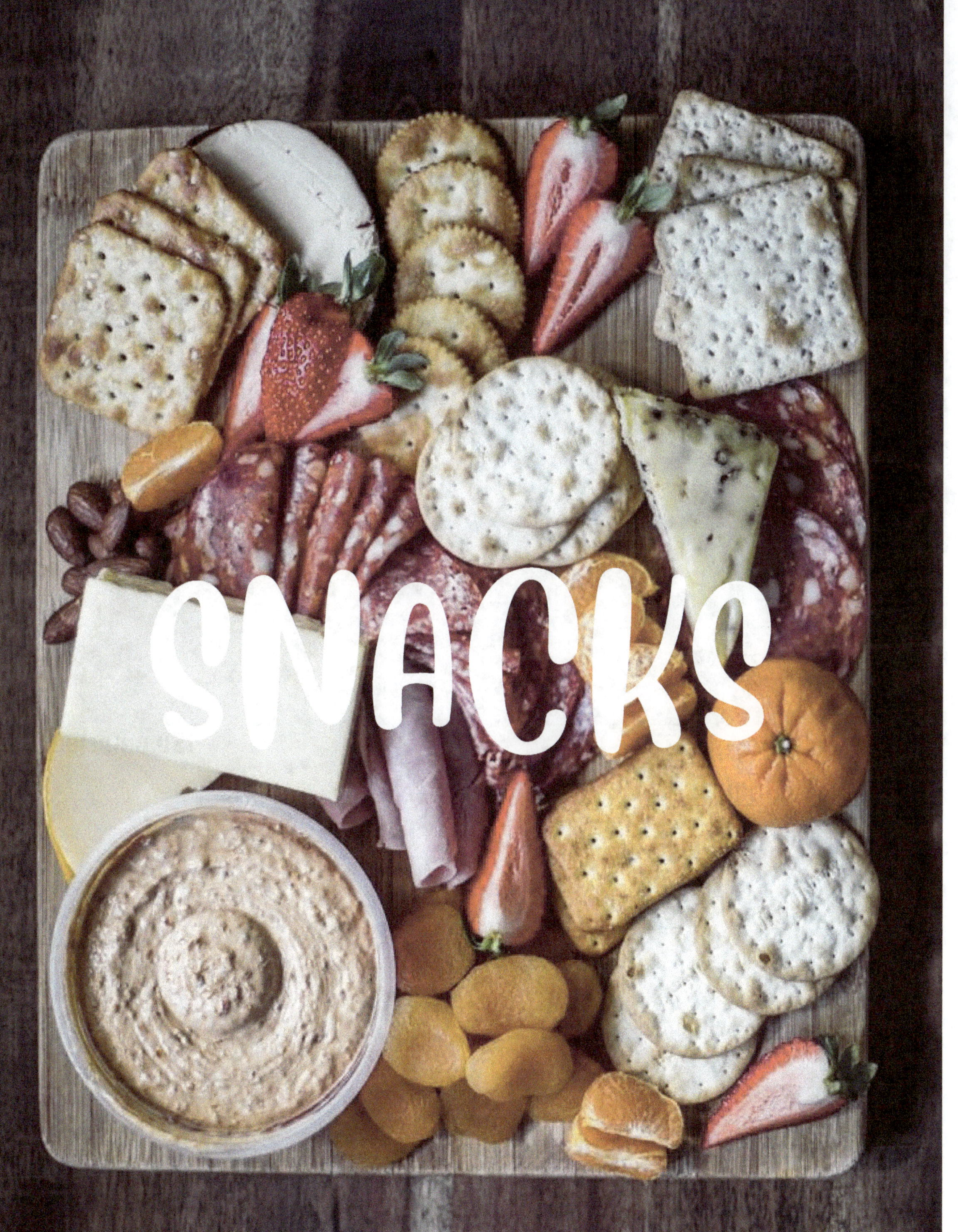

SNACKS

GREEK YOGURT WITH HONEY AND BERRIES

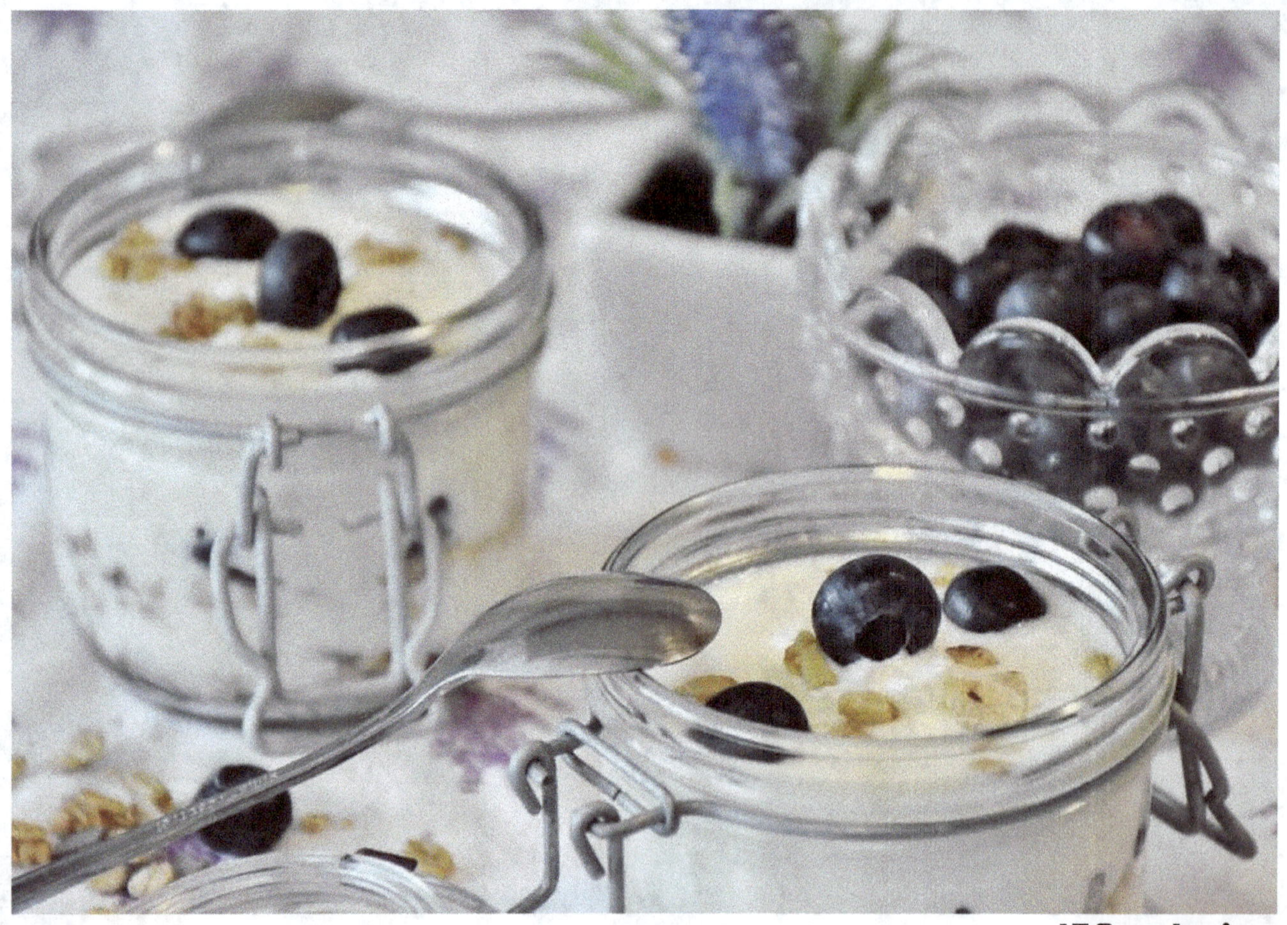

150 calories

What You'll Need:

- 1 cup Greek yogurt

- 1 tbsp. honey

- ½ cup mixed berries (e.g., strawberries, blueberries, raspberries)

Directions:

- Spoon Greek yogurt into a bowl.

- Drizzle honey over the yogurt.

- Top with mixed berries.

ALMONDS AND DRIED FRUIT MIX

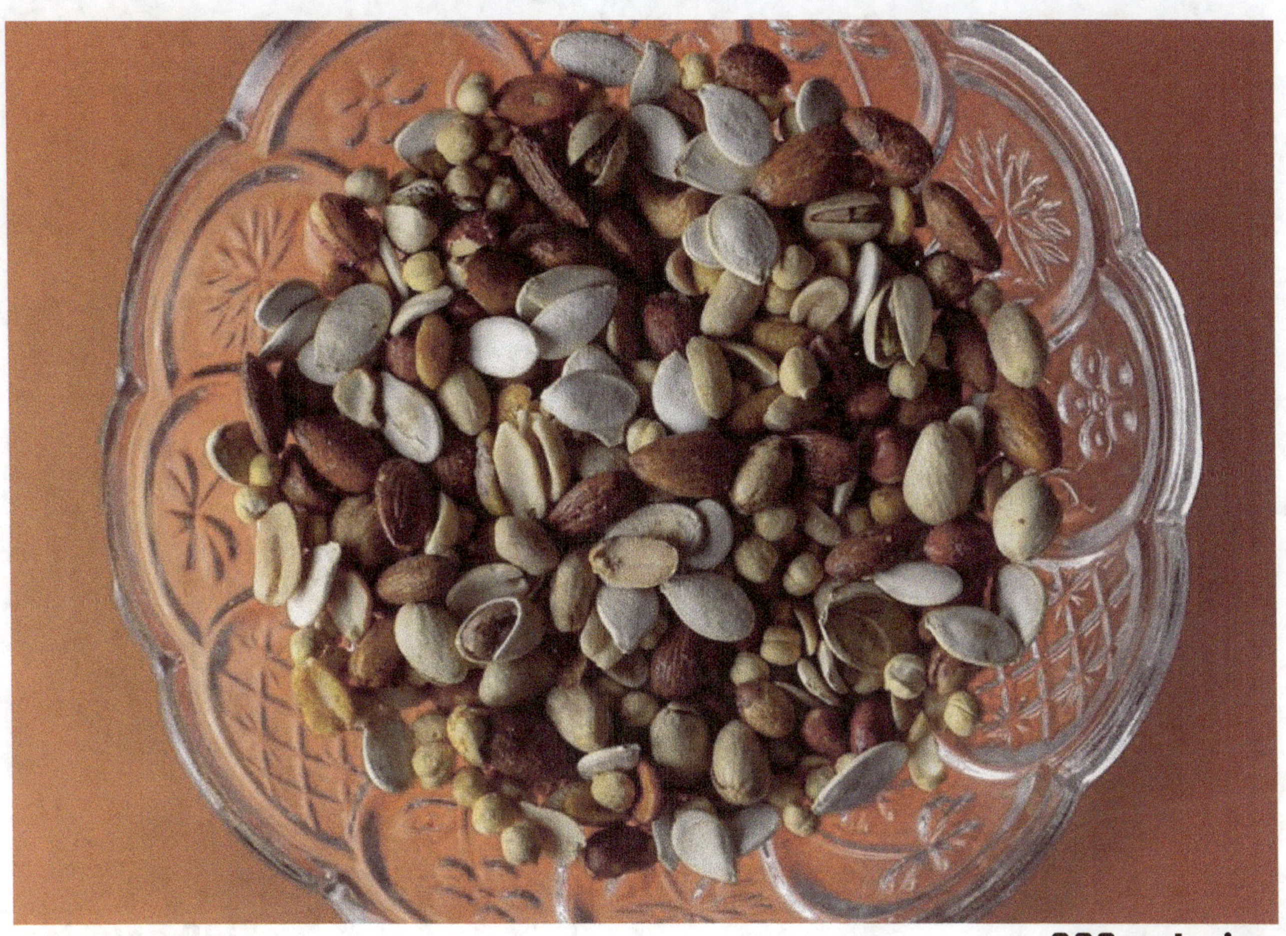

200 calories

What You'll Need:

- ¼ cup almonds

- ¼ cup dried fruit (e.g., raisins, apricots, cranberries)

Directions:

- Combine almonds and dried fruit in a bowl.

- Mix well and serve

APPLE SLICES WITH PEANUT BUTTER

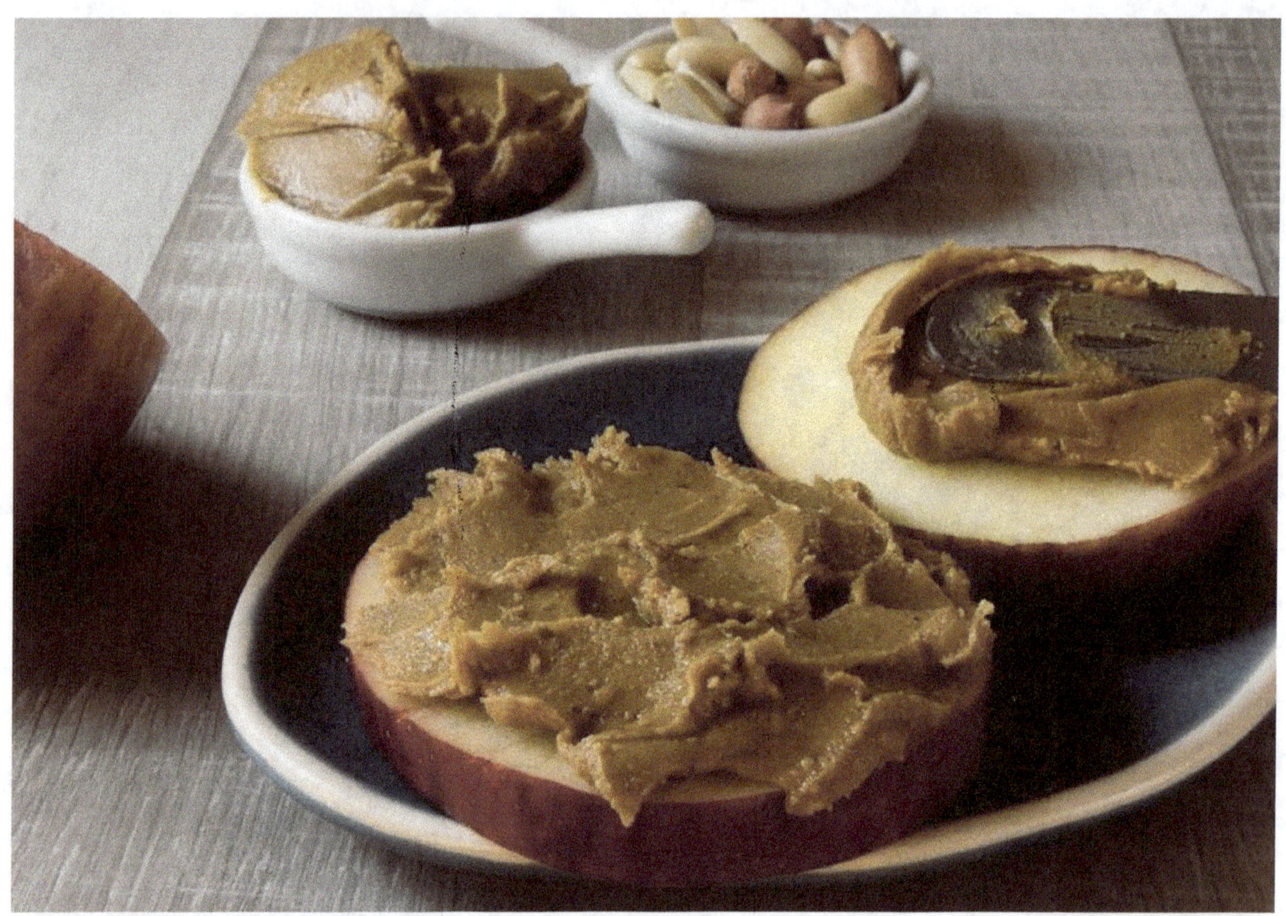

180 calories

What You'll Need:

- 1 medium apple

- 2 tbsp peanut butter

Directions:

- Slice the apple into wedges.

- Serve with peanut butter for dipping

VEGGIE STICKS WITH HUMMUS

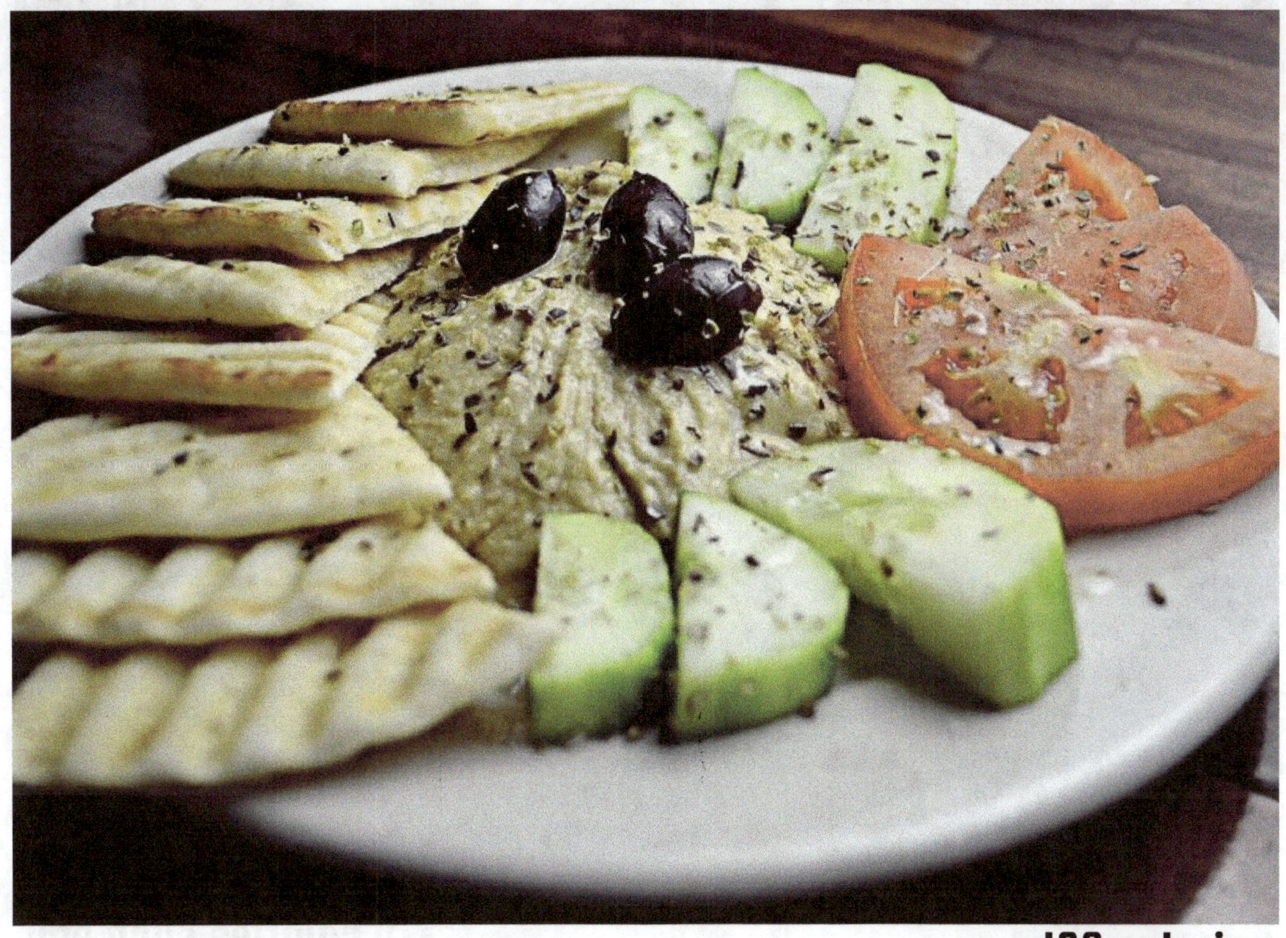

120 calories

What You'll Need:

- 1 cup assorted veggie sticks (e.g., carrots, celery, bell peppers)
- ¼ cup hummus

Directions:

- Arrange veggie sticks on a plate.
- Serve with hummus for dipping

HARD-BOILED EGGS

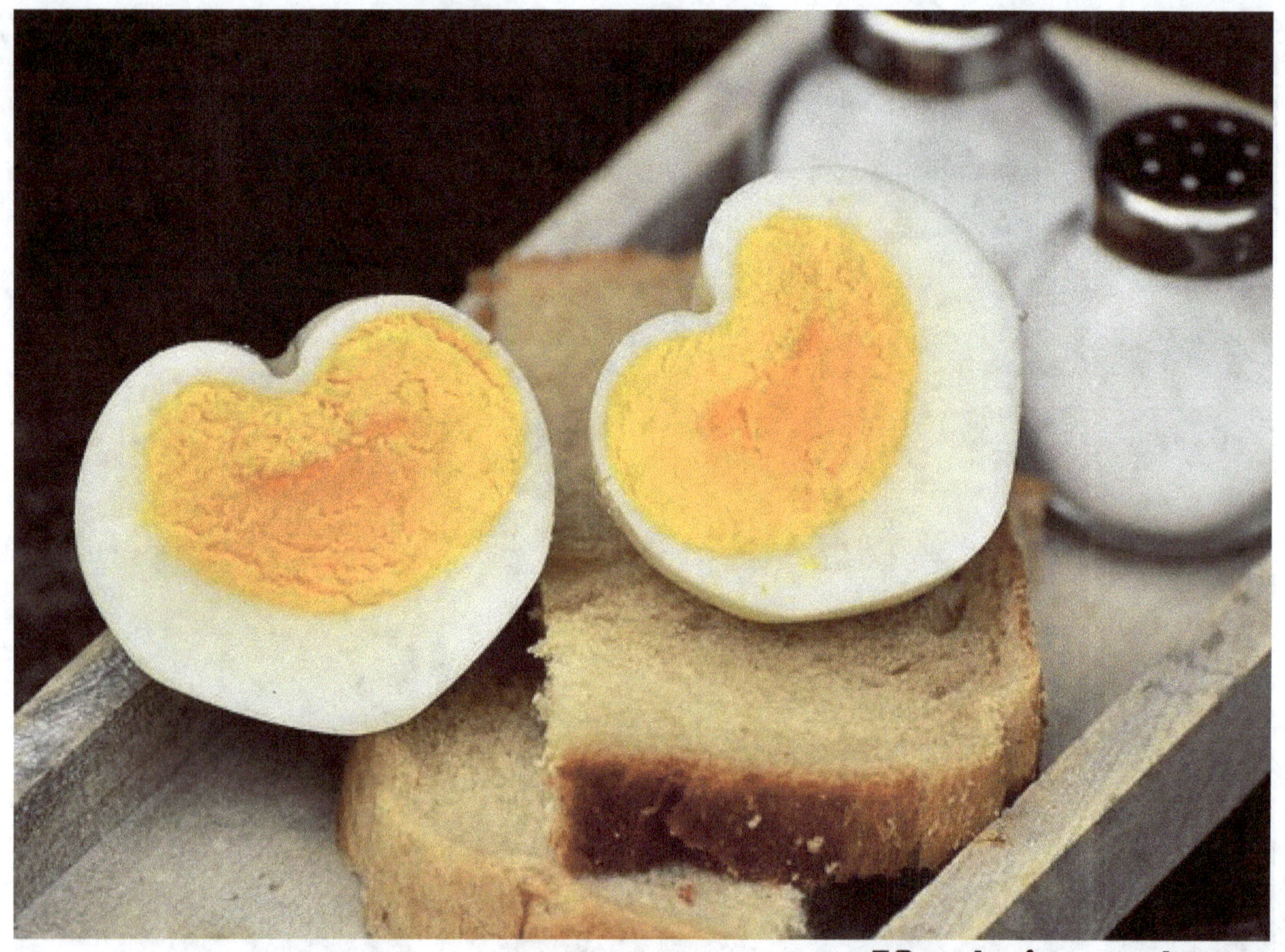

70 calories each egg

<u>**What You'll Need:**</u>

- **1 egg**

<u>**Directions:**</u>

- **Place eggs in a pot and cover with water.**

- **Bring to a boil, then reduce heat and simmer for 9-12 minutes.**

- **Cool in ice water, peel, and serve.**

AIR-POPPED POPCORN

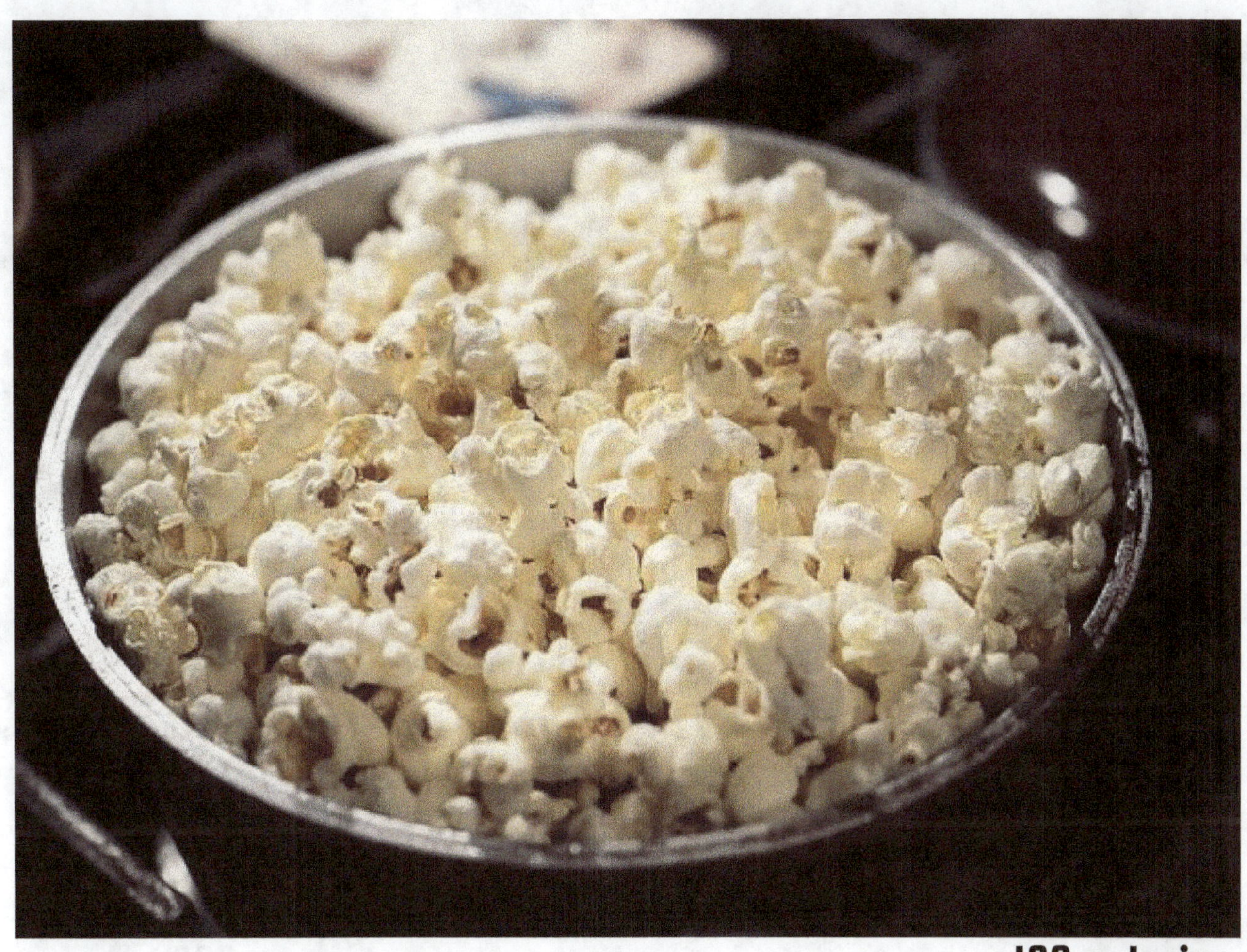

100 calories

<u>**What You'll Need:**</u>

- 3 cups air-popped popcorn

<u>**Directions:**</u>

- Pop popcorn according to your air popper's instructions.

- Serve plain or with a light seasoning of your choice

CHEESE AND WHOLE GRAIN CRACKERS

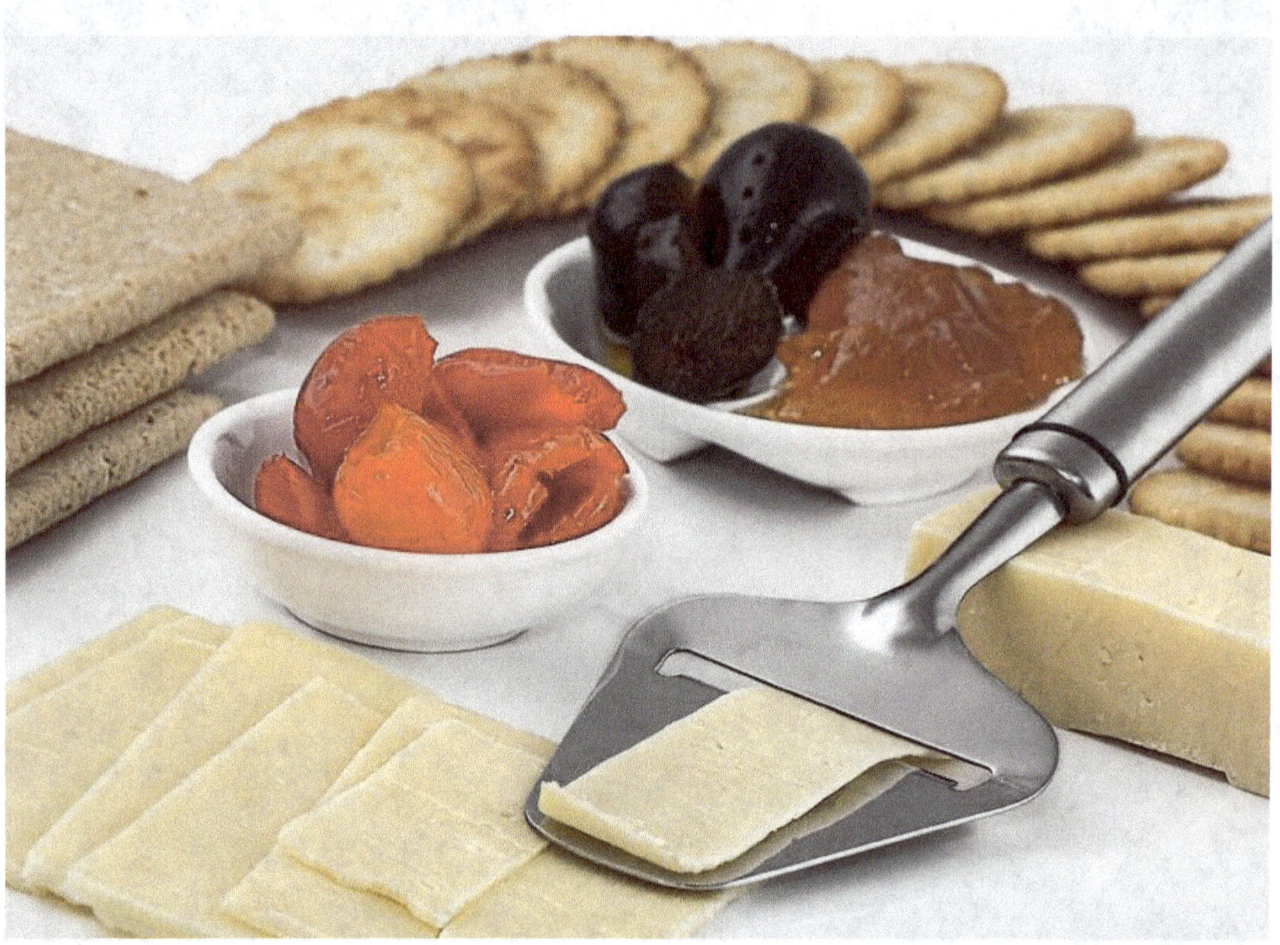

200 calories

<u>**What You'll Need:**</u>

- 1 oz cheese (e.g., cheddar, mozzarella)
- 6 whole grain crackers

<u>**Directions:**</u>

- Slice cheese into small pieces.
- Serve with whole grain crackers.

EDAMAME

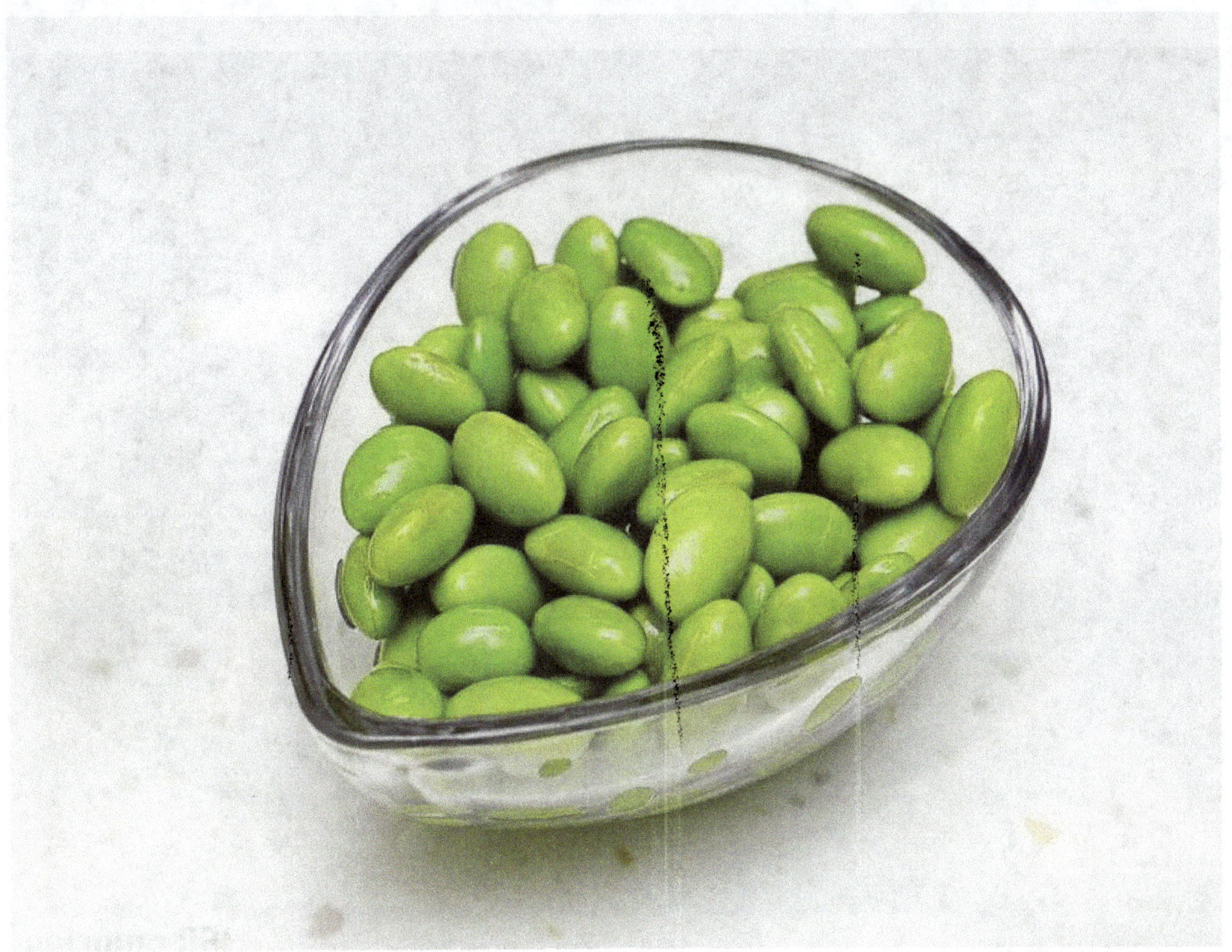

120 calories

What You'll Need:

- 1 cup edamame (shelled or in the pod)

Directions:

- Steam or boil edamame until tender.

- Sprinkle with a pinch of salt and serve.

FRUIT SALAD

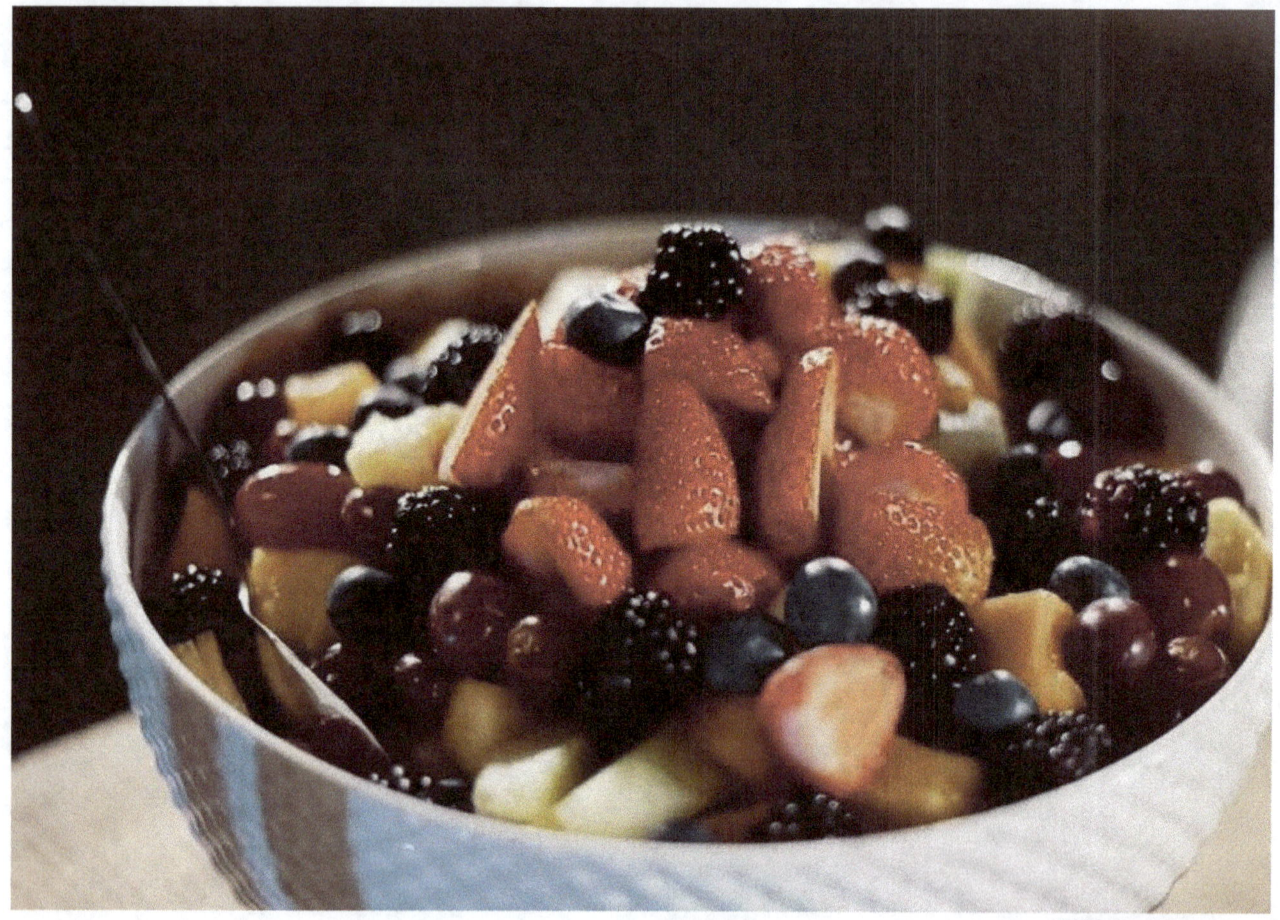

150 calories

What You'll Need:

- 1 cup mixed fruit (e.g., melon, berries, grapes, apple)

Directions:

- Chop the fruit into bite-sized pieces.
- Mix together in a bowl and serve.

DARK CHOCOLATE

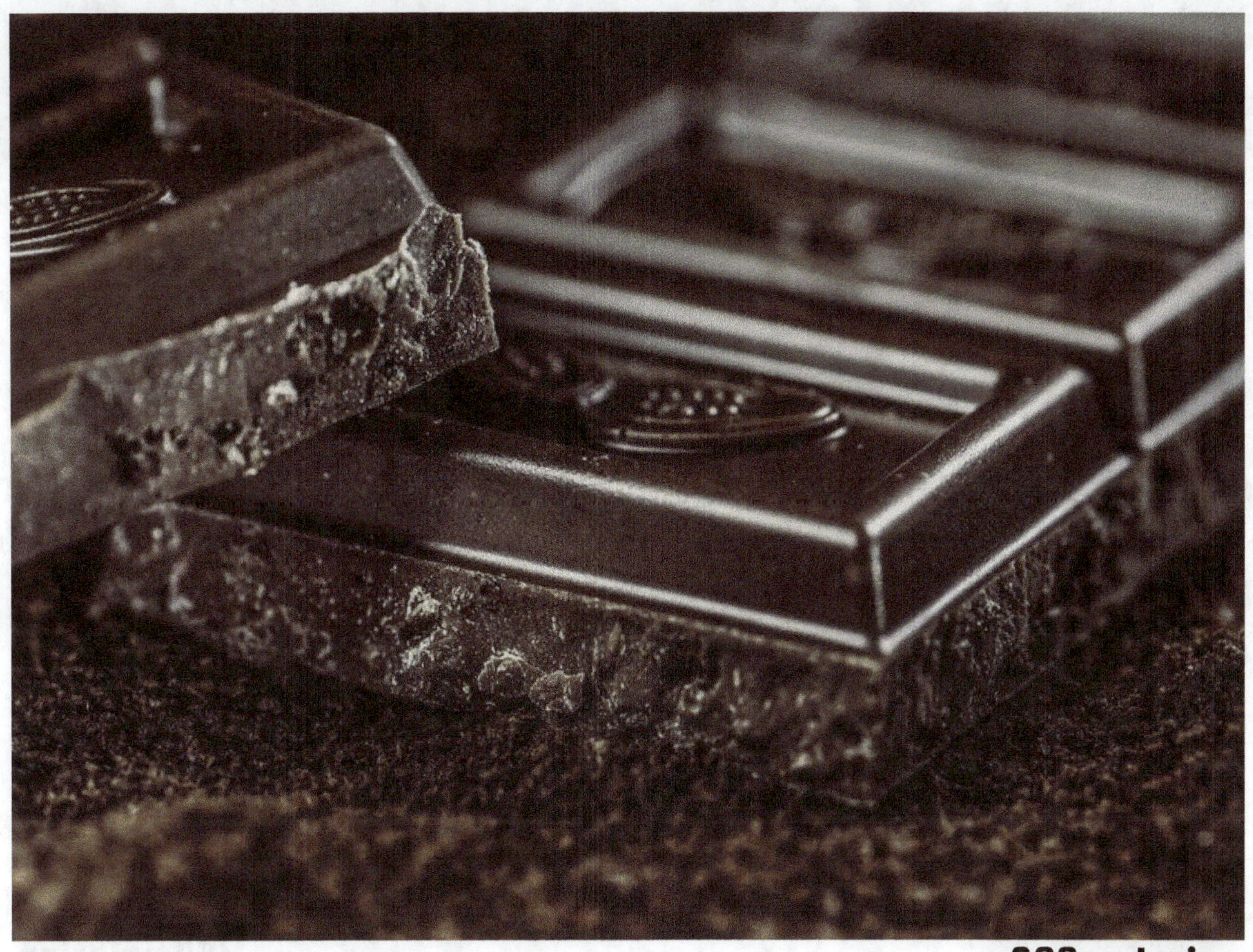

200 calories

<u>**What You'll Need:**</u>

- 1 oz dark chocolate (70% cocoa or higher)

<u>**Directions:**</u>

- Break the chocolate into pieces.

- Enjoy as a simple, satisfying snack.

CUCUMBER SLICES WITH TZATZIKI

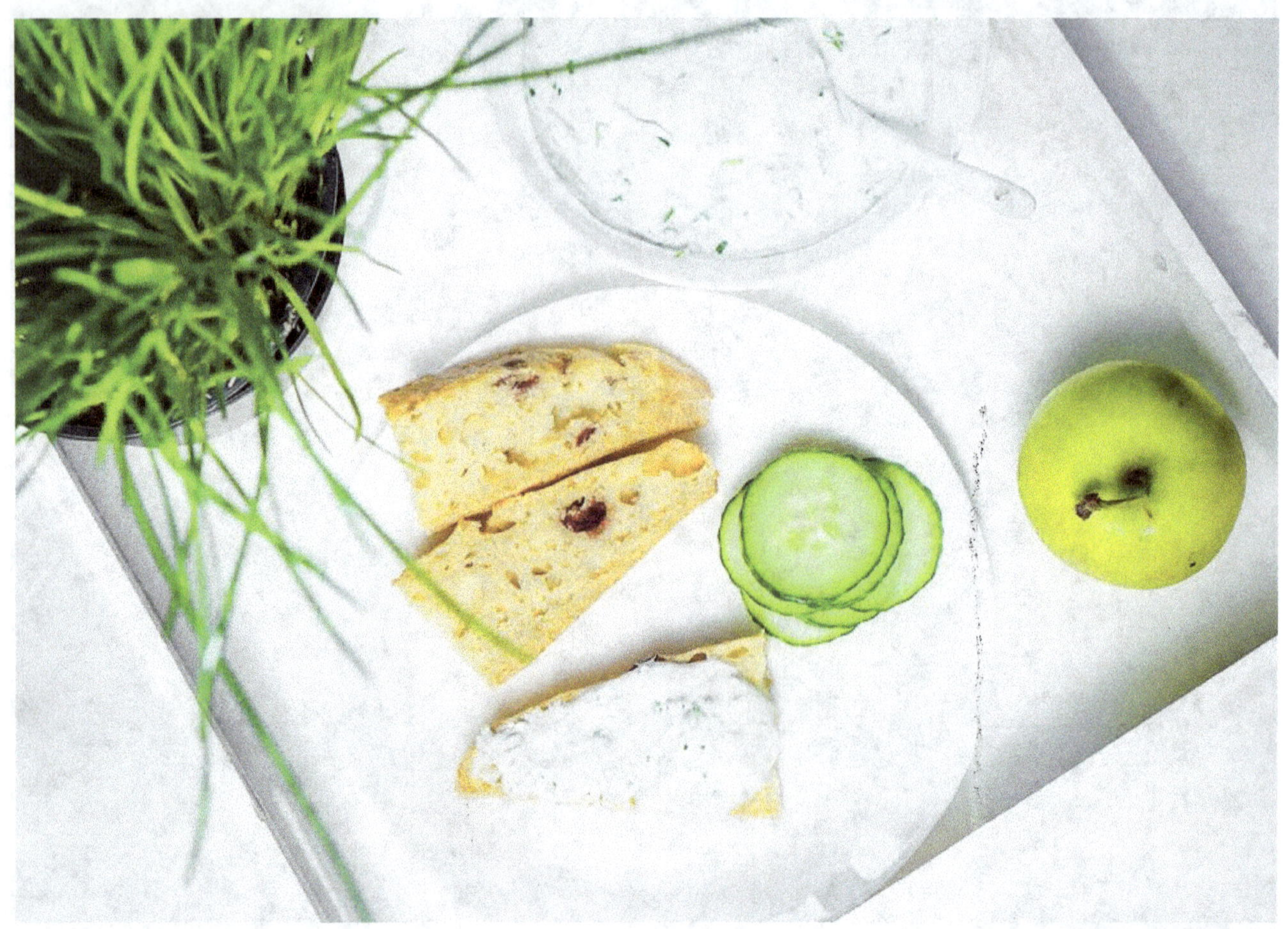

100 calories

What You'll Need:

- 1 cucumber
- ¼ cup tzatziki sauce

Directions:

- Slice cucumber into rounds.
- Serve with tzatziki sauce for dipping.

SWEET POTATO CHIPS

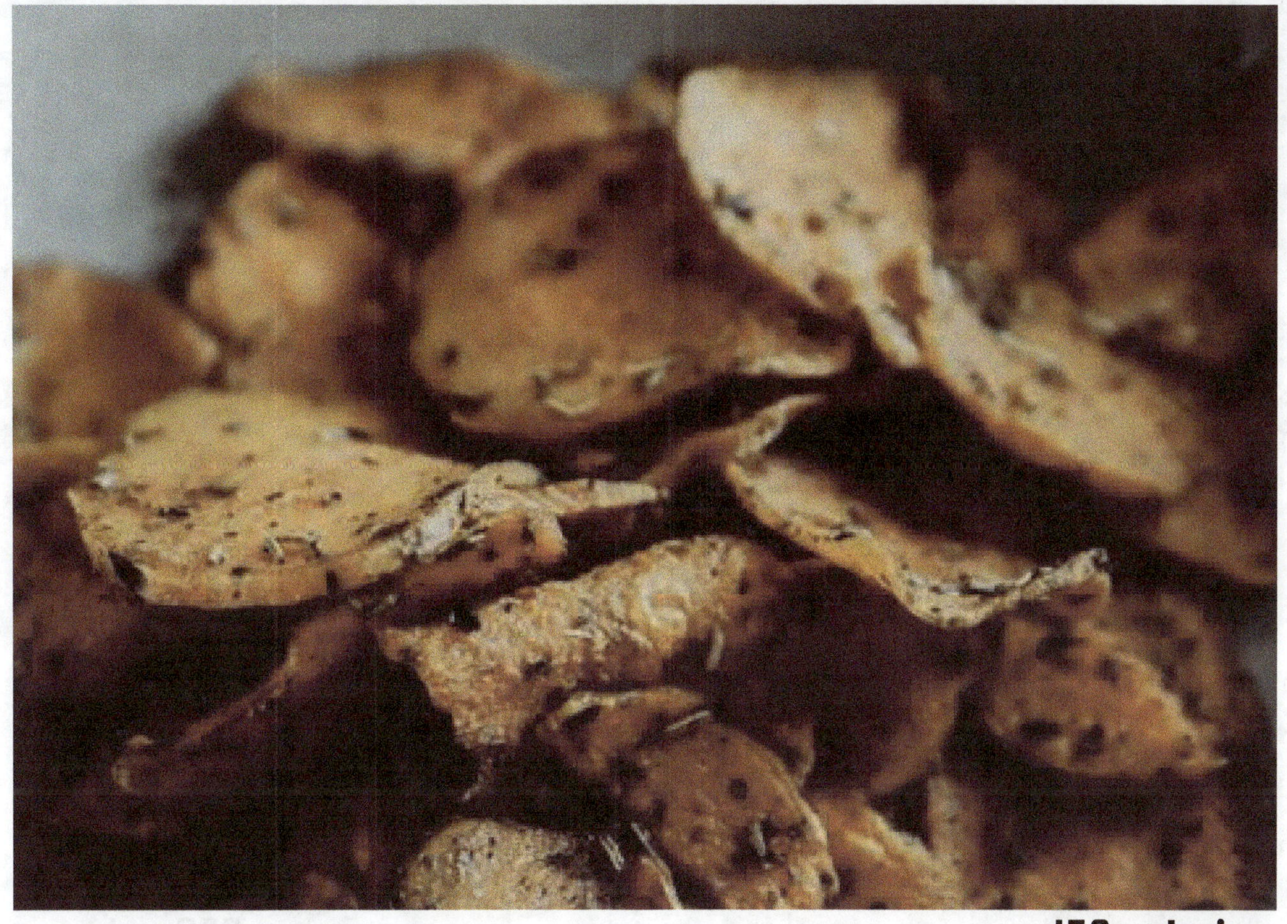

150 calories

<u>**What You'll Need:**</u>

- 1 large, sweet potato

- 1 tbsp olive oil

- Salt and pepper to taste

<u>**Directions:**</u>

- Preheat oven to 400°F (200°C).
- Slice sweet potato thinly.
- Toss with olive oil, salt, and pepper.
- Arrange on a baking sheet and bake for 15–20 minutes, or until crispy.

PROTEIN BARS

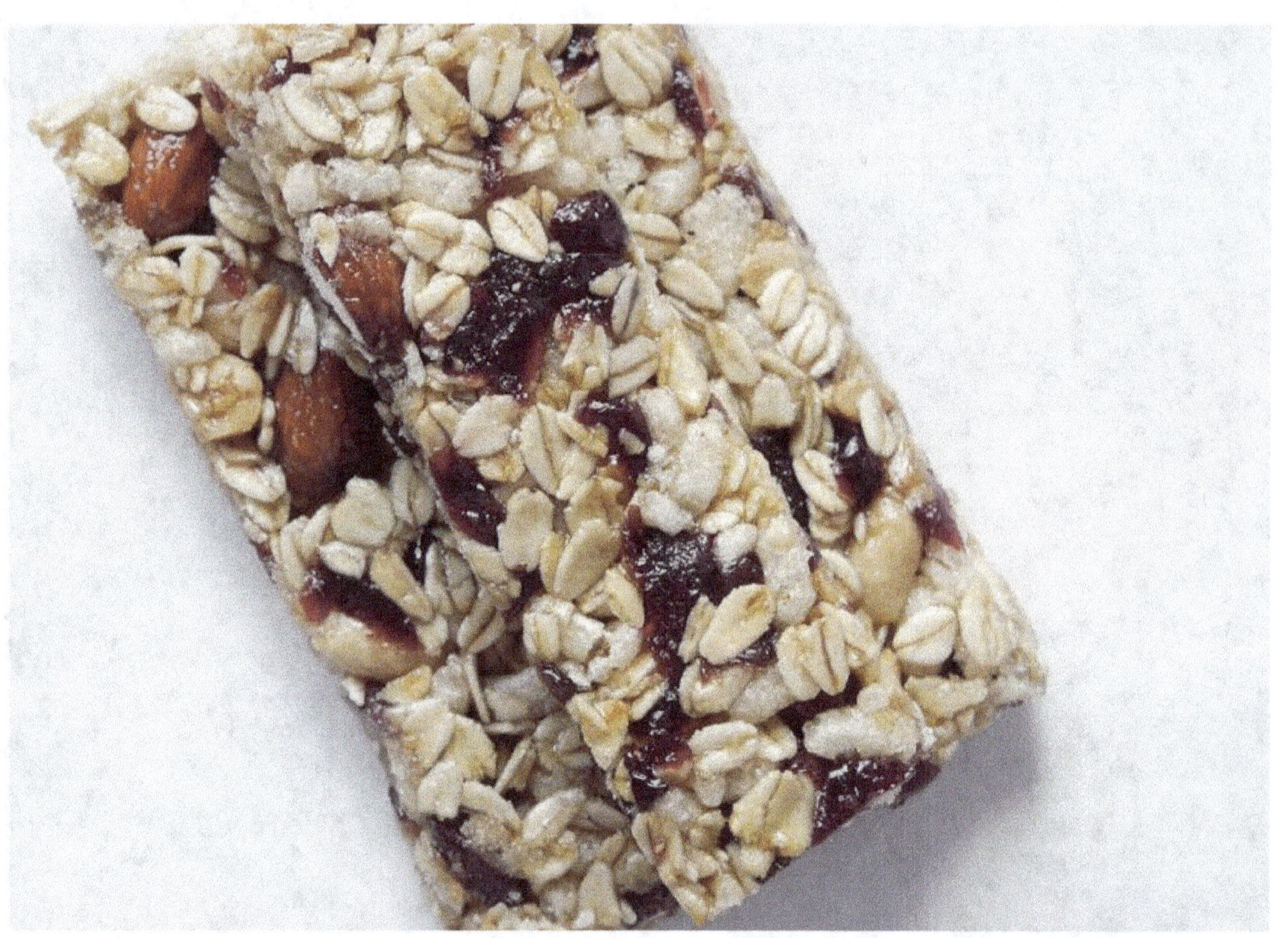

200 calories

<u>**What You'll Need:**</u>

- **1 protein bar (store-bought or homemade)**

<u>**Directions:**</u>

- **Simply unwrap the protein bar and enjoy.**

FRUIT AND NUT MIX

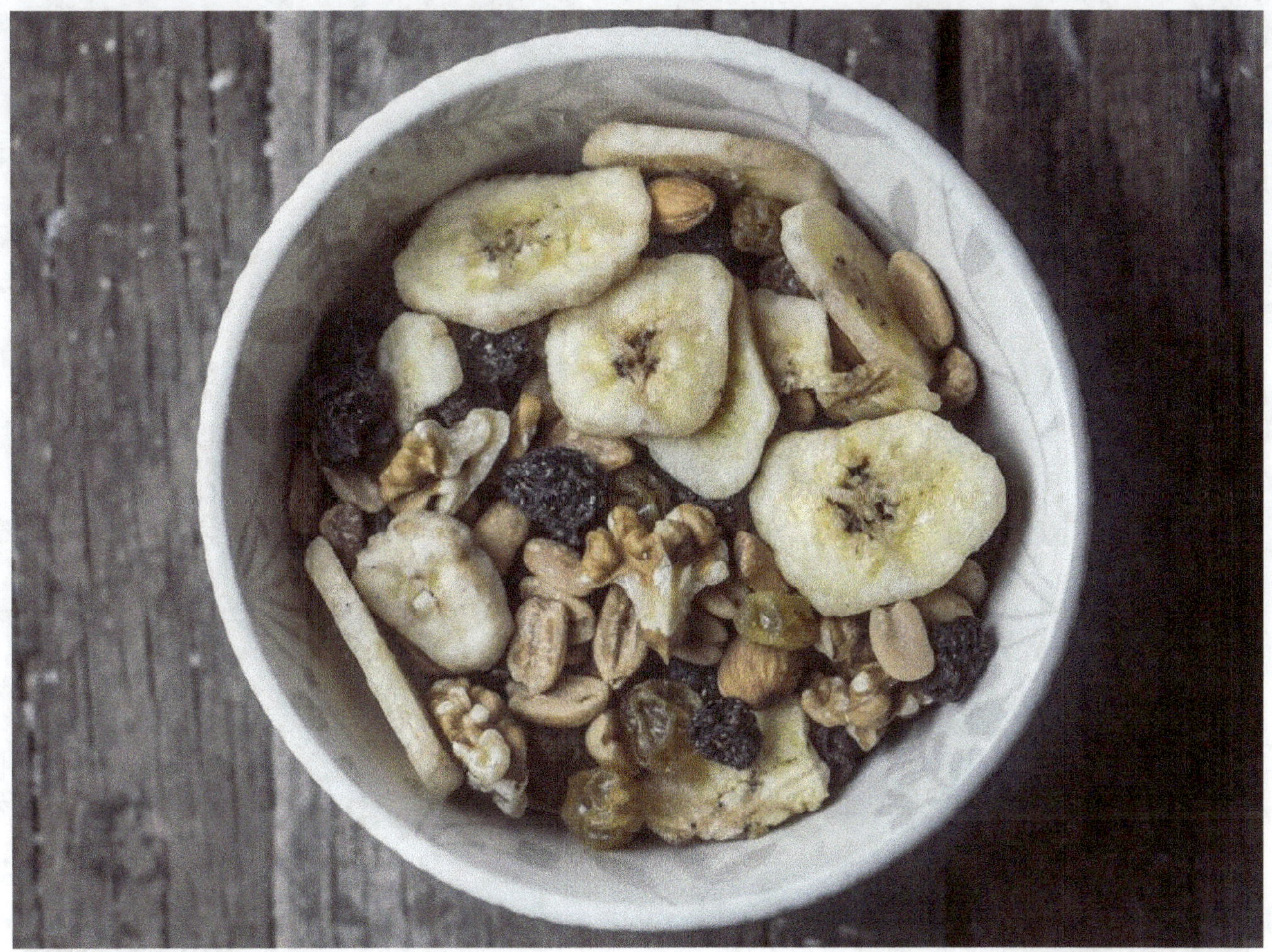

180 calories

<u>**What You'll Need:**</u>

- ¼ cup mixed nuts (almonds, walnuts, cashews)

- ¼ cup dried fruit (raisins, cranberries, apricots)

<u>Directions:</u>

- Combine nuts and dried fruit in a bowl.
- Mix well and serve.

RICE CAKES WITH AVOCADO

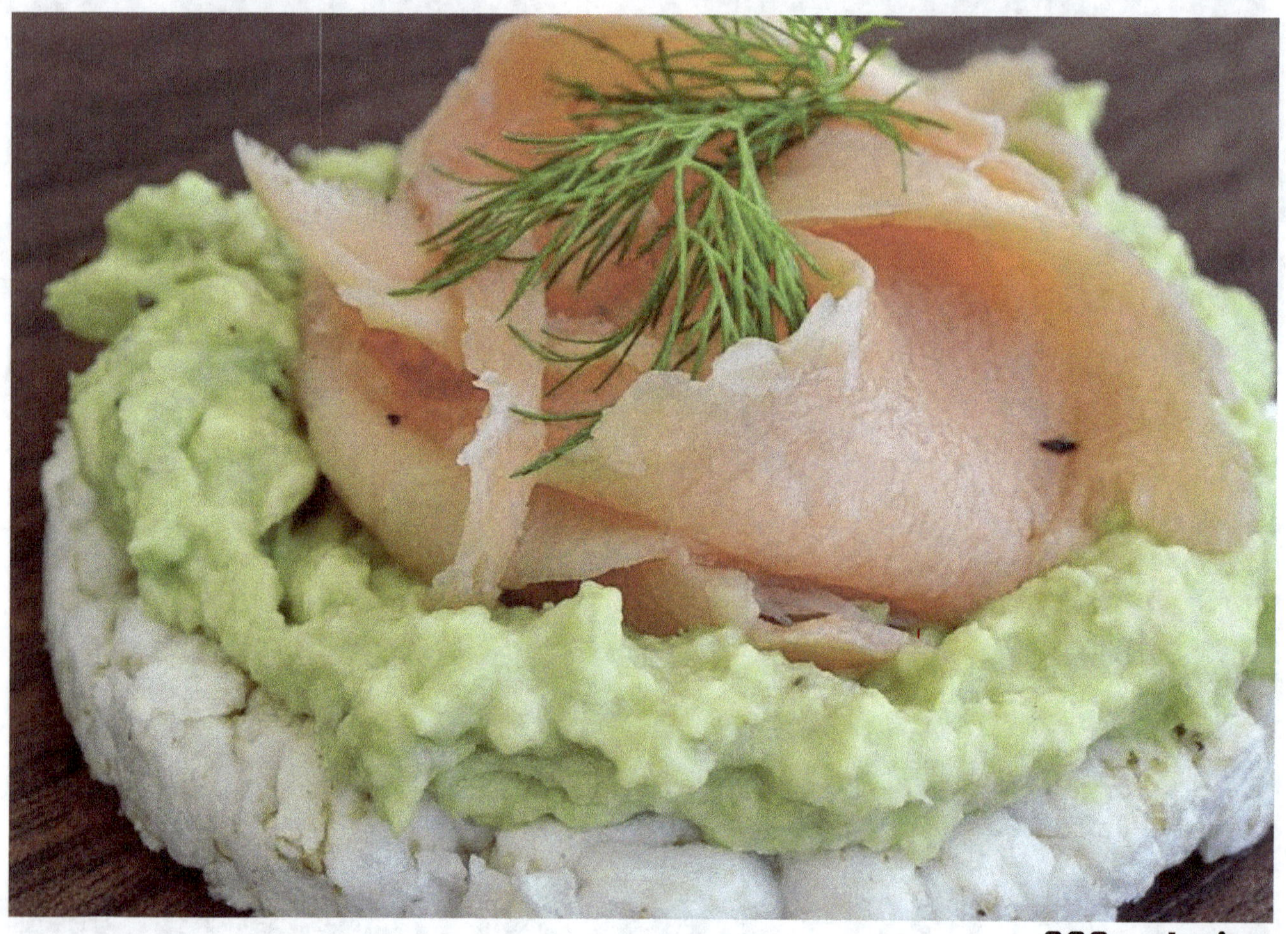

200 calories

What You'll Need:

- 2 rice cakes
- ½ avocado
- Salt and pepper to taste

Directions:

- Mash avocado and spread it on the rice cakes.
- Season with salt and pepper.

BAKED APPLE CHIPS

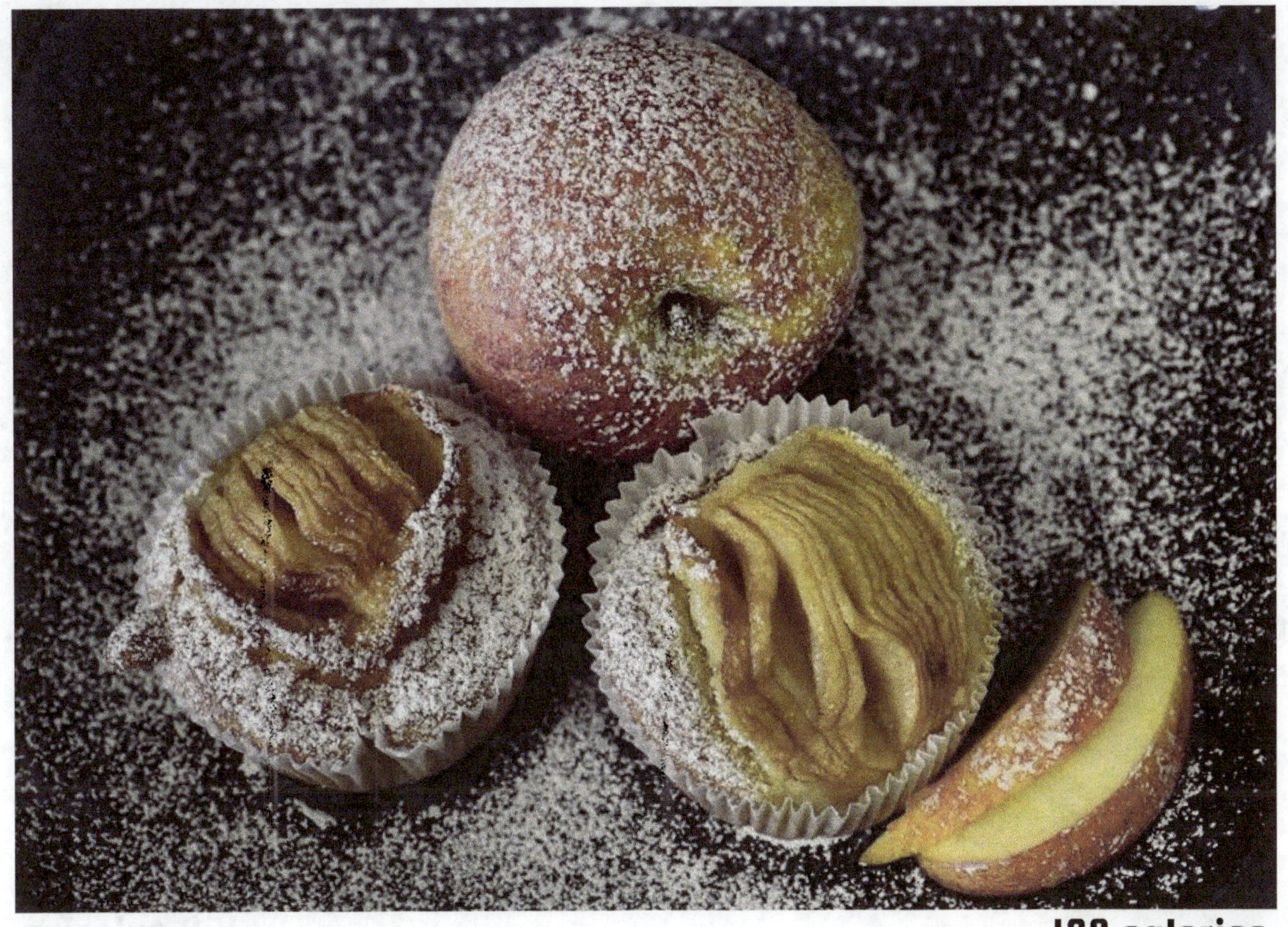

What You'll Need:

- 1 apple
- ½ tsp cinnamon

Directions:

- Preheat oven to 275°F (135°C).
- Slice apple thinly.
- Arrange slices on a baking sheet and sprinkle with cinnamon.
- Bake for 1 hour, turning halfway through, until crisp

COTTAGE CHEESE WITH PINEAPPLE

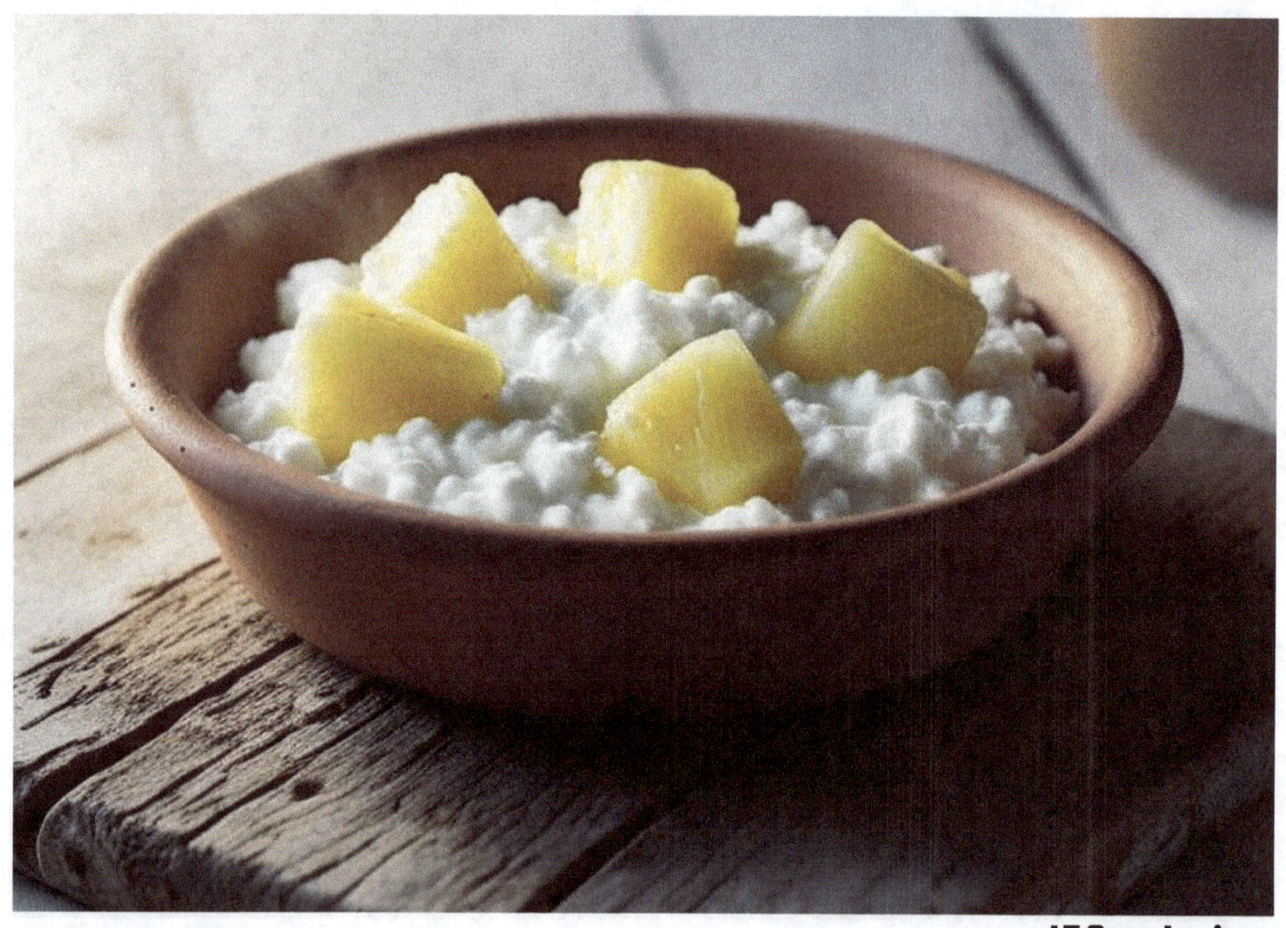

150 calories

What You'll Need:

- ½ cup cottage cheese
- ½ cup pineapple chunks

Directions:

- Mix cottage cheese with pineapple chunks.
- Serve chilled.

CARROT AND CELERY STICKS

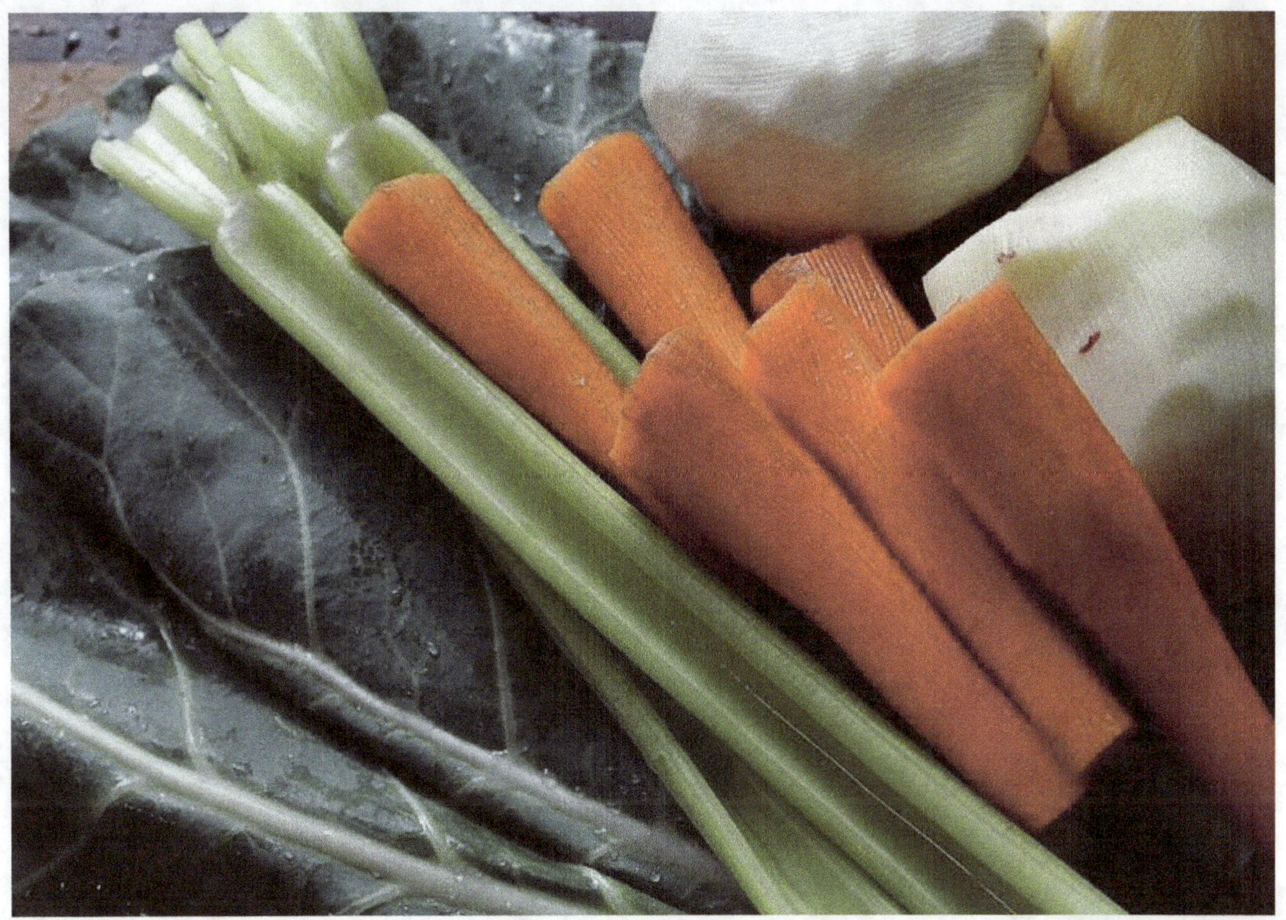

100 calories

<u>**What You'll Need:**</u>

- **1 cup carrot sticks**

- **1 cup celery sticks**

<u>**Directions:**</u>

- **Arrange carrot and celery sticks on a plate.**

- **Serve as a snack**

YOGURT PARFAIT

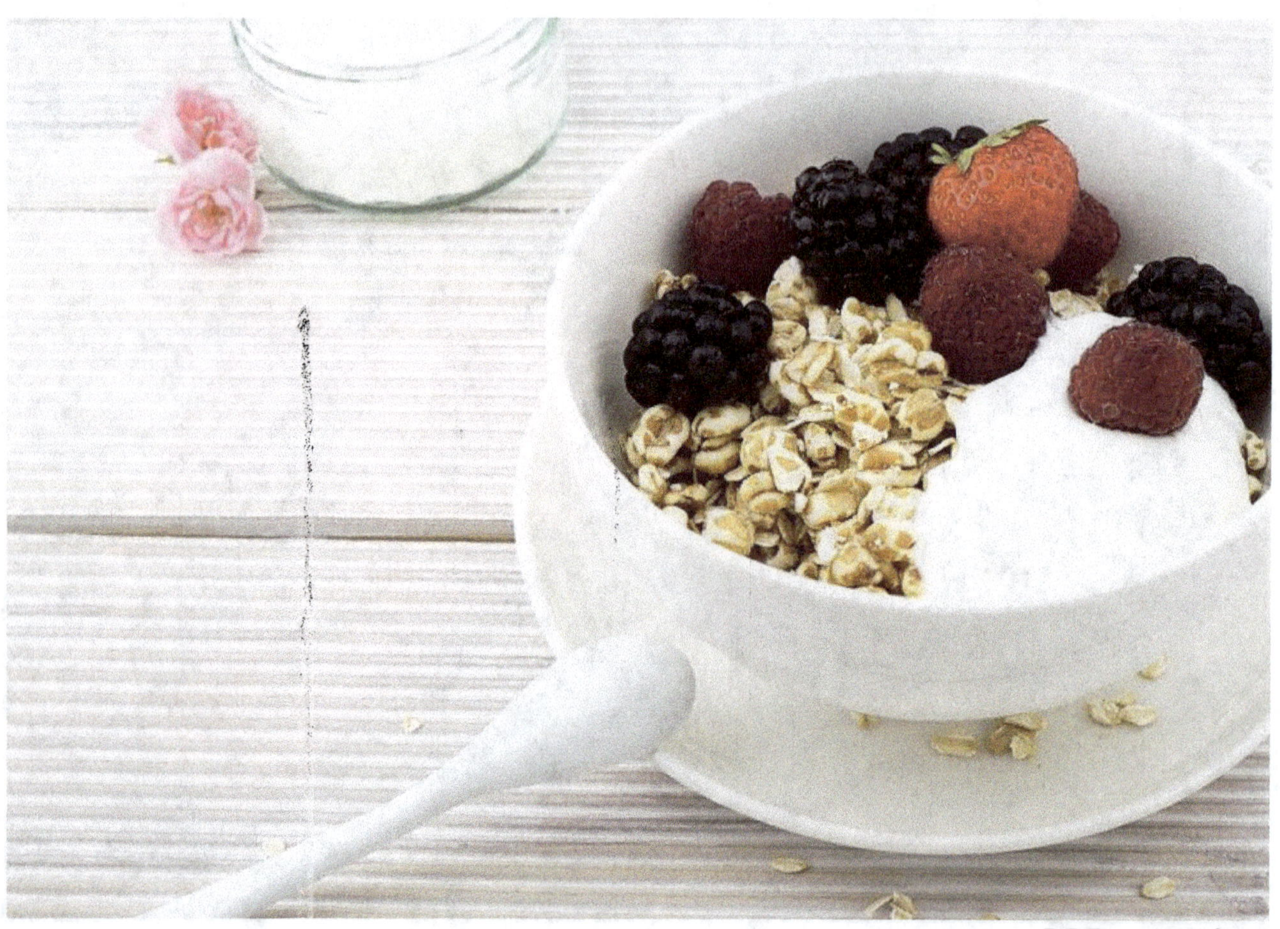

200 calories

What You'll Need:

- 1 cup Greek yogurt
- ¼ cup granola
- ¼ cup mixed berries

Directions:

- Layer Greek yogurt, granola, and mixed berries in a glass.
- Serve immediately.

FROZEN GRAPES

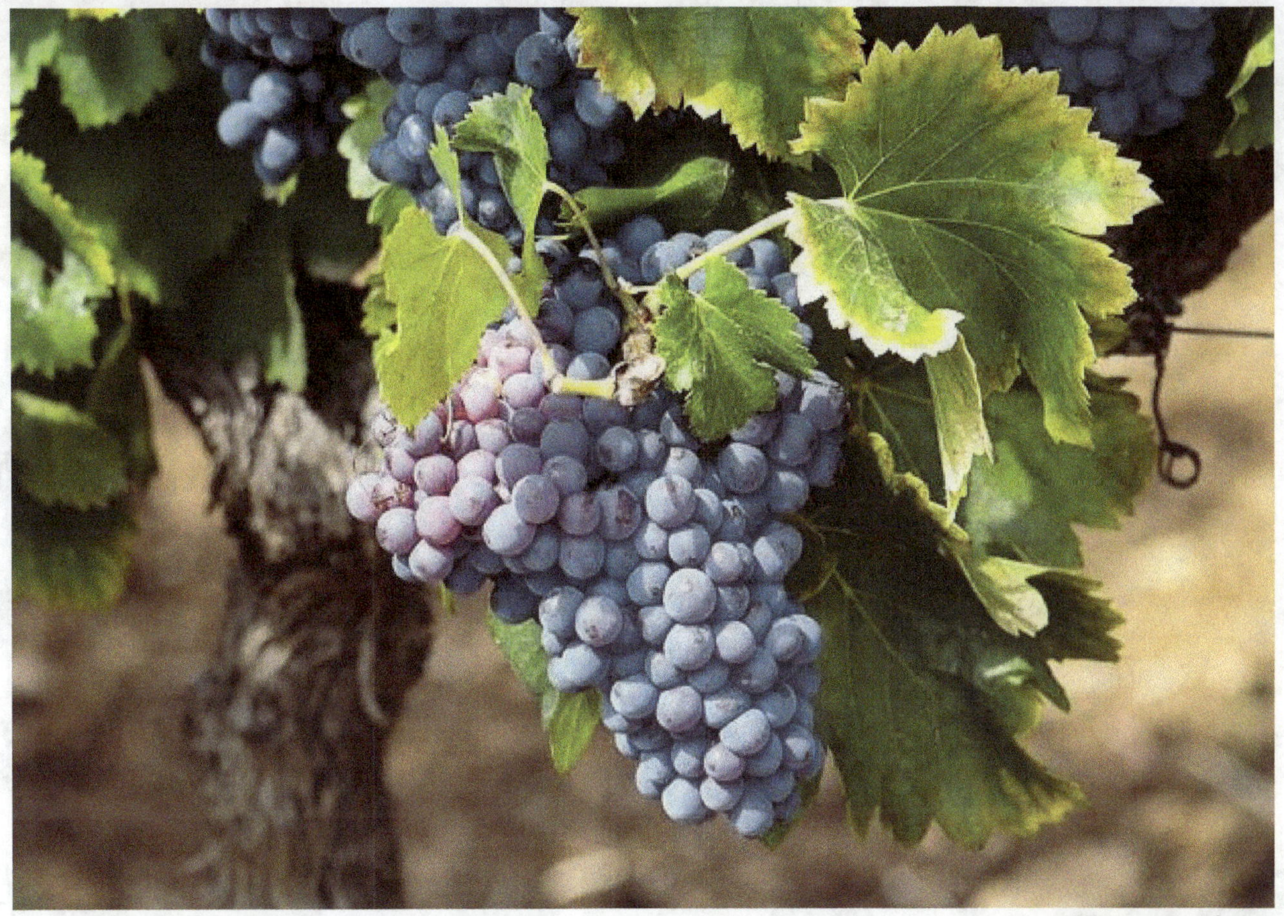

100 calories

<u>**What You'll Need:**</u>

- 1 cup grapes

<u>**Directions:**</u>

- Wash and dry grapes.

- Freeze for at least 2 hours.

- Serve frozen.

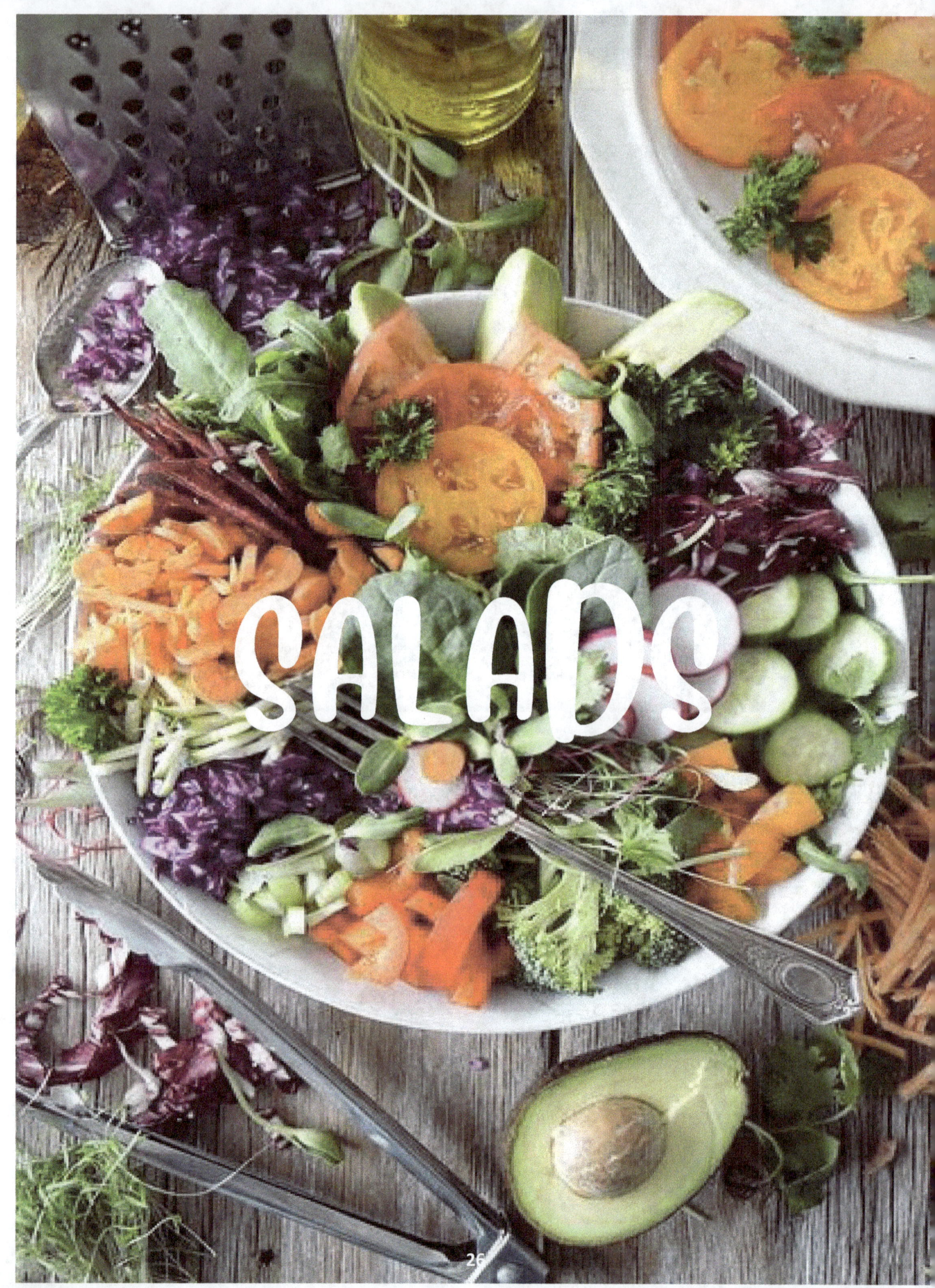
SALADS

CLASSIC CAESAR SALAD

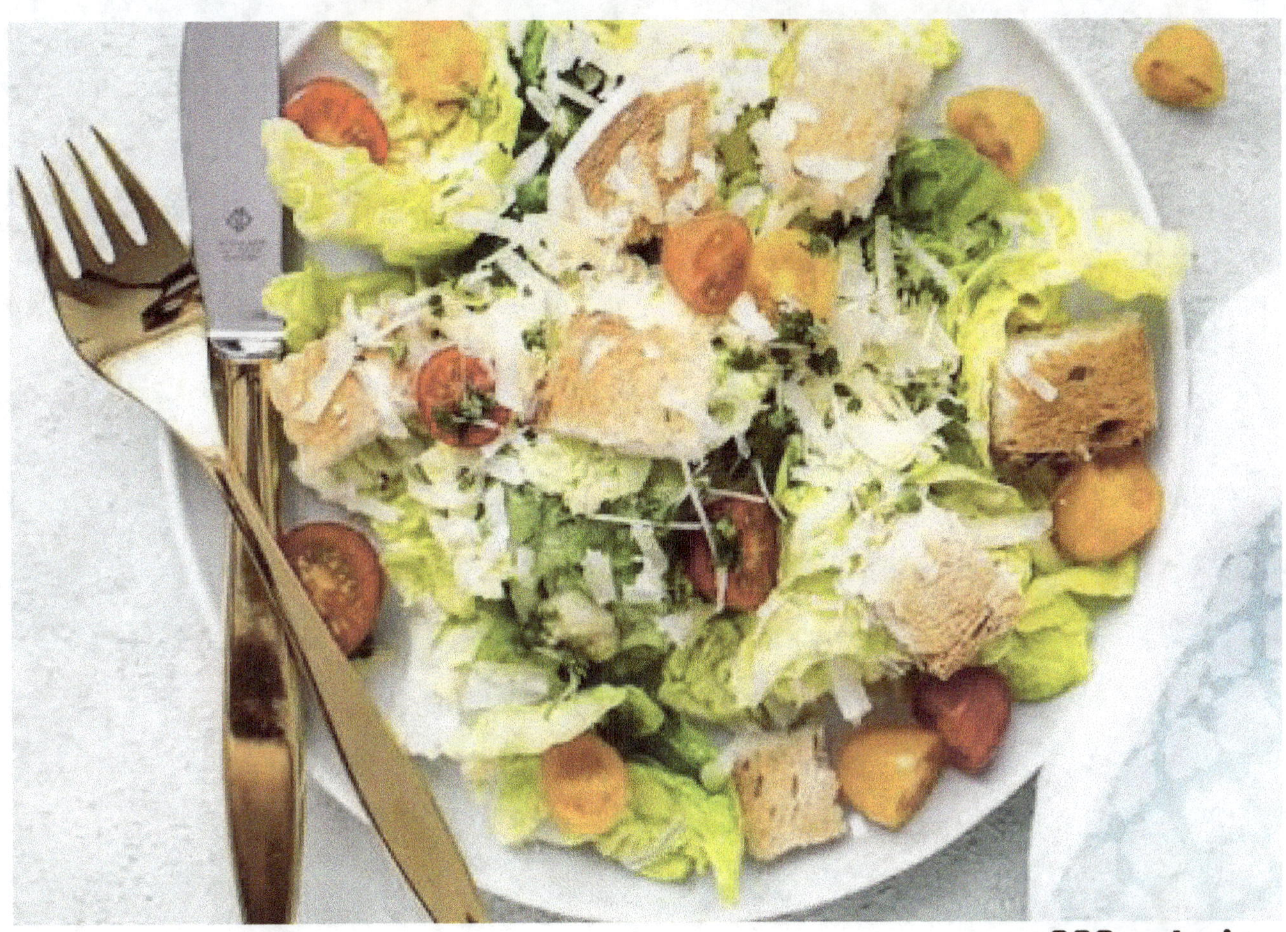

300 calories

What You'll Need:

- 2 cups romaine lettuce
- ¼ cup Caesar dressing
- ¼ cup grated Parmesan cheese
- ½ cup croutons

Directions:

- Tear romaine lettuce into bite-sized pieces and place in a bowl.
- Toss with Caesar dressing.
- Top with Parmesan cheese and croutons.

GREEK SALAD

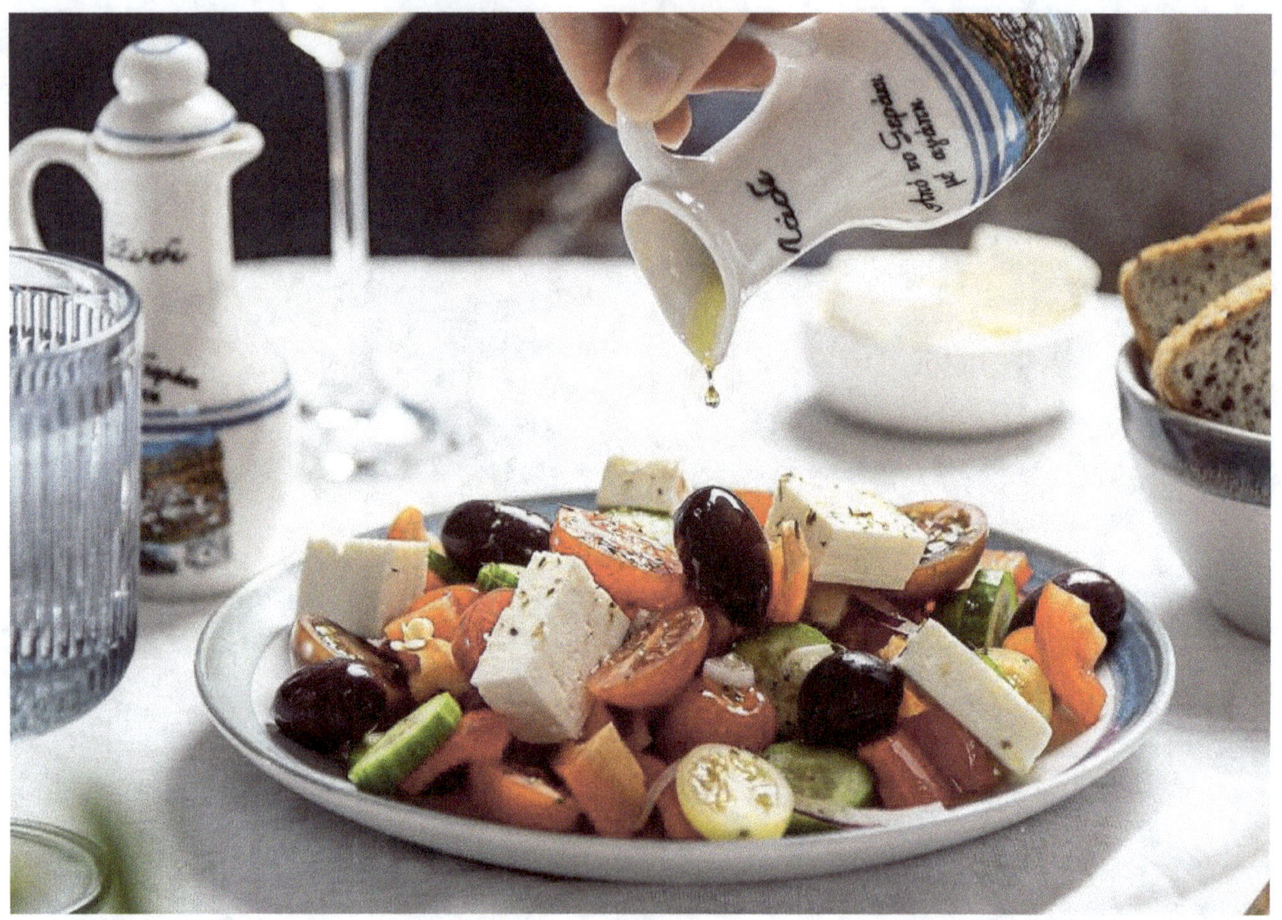

250 calories

What You'll Need:

- 1 cup cucumber, diced
- 1 cup tomatoes, diced
- ¼ cup Kalamata olives
- ¼ cup feta cheese, crumbled
- 2 tbsp olive oil
- 1 tbsp red wine vinegar
- 1 tsp dried oregano

Directions:

- Combine cucumber, tomatoes, olives, and feta cheese in a bowl.
- Drizzle with olive oil.
- Sprinkle with dried oregano and toss gently.

QUINOA AND BLACK BEAN SALAD

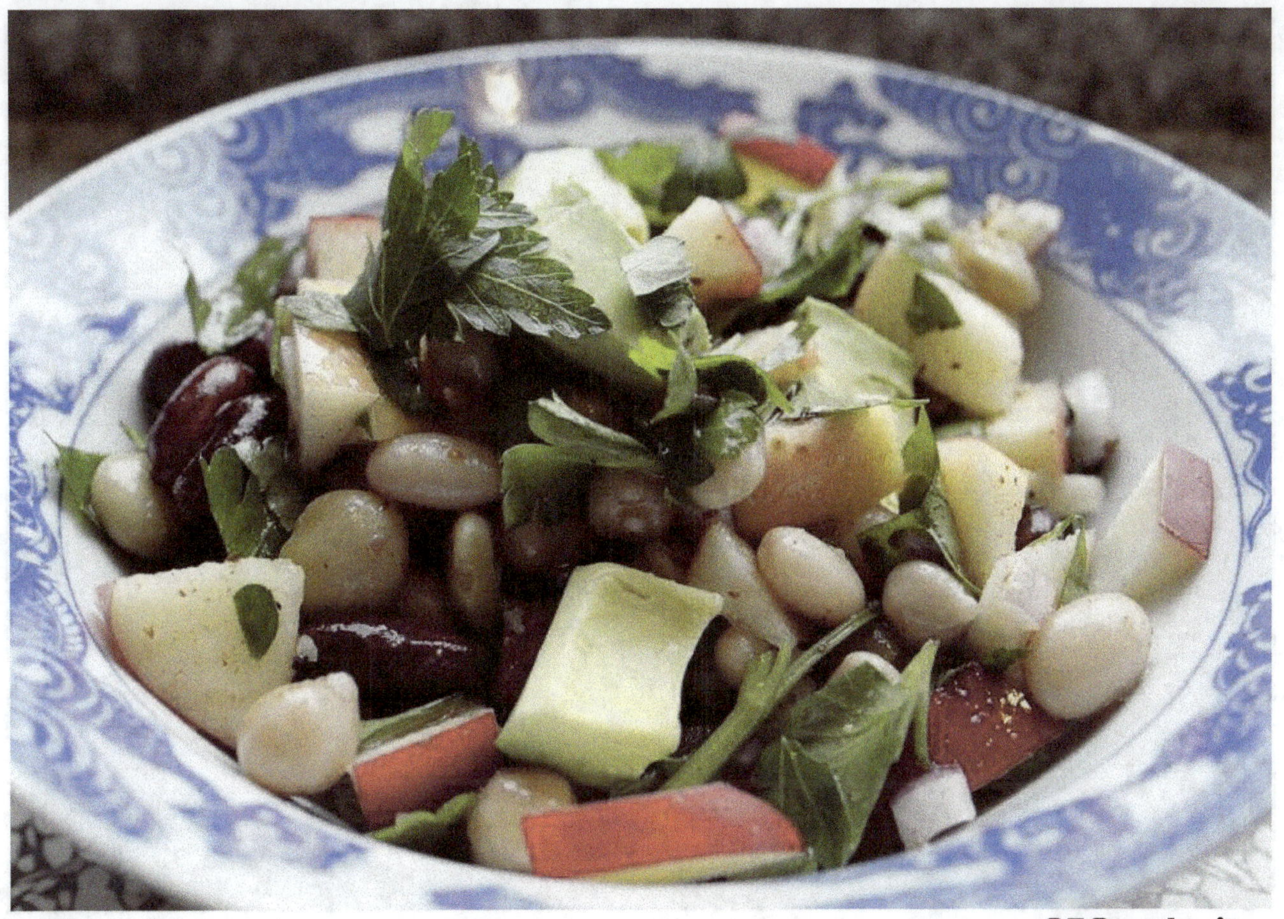

350 calories

What You'll Need:

- 1 cup cooked quinoa
- ½ cup black beans, drained and rinsed
- ½ cup corn kernels
- ¼ cup chopped cilantro
- 2 tbsp lime juice
- 1 tbsp olive oil

Directions:

- Combine quinoa, black beans, corn, and cilantro in a bowl.
- Drizzle with lime juice and olive oil.
- Toss well and serve.

SPINACH AND STRAWBERRY SALAD

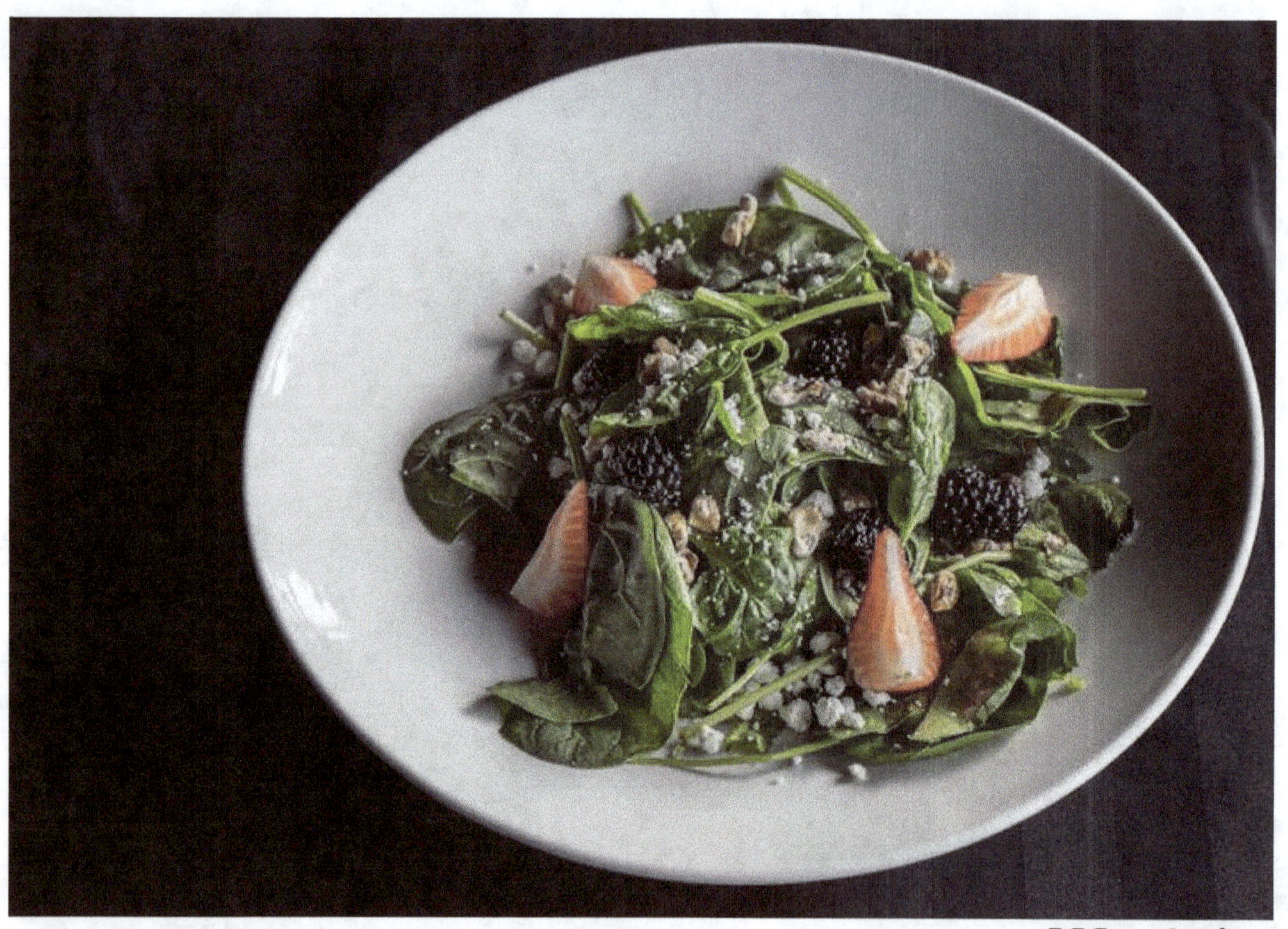

200 calories

<u>**What You'll Need:**</u>

- **2 cups fresh spinach**

- **½ cup sliced strawberries**

- **¼ cup sliced almonds**

- **2 tbsp balsamic vinaigrette**

<u>**Directions:**</u>

- **Place spinach in a bowl.**

- **Top with strawberries and almonds.**

- **Drizzle with balsamic vinaigrette and toss gently**

KALE AND AVOCADO SALAD

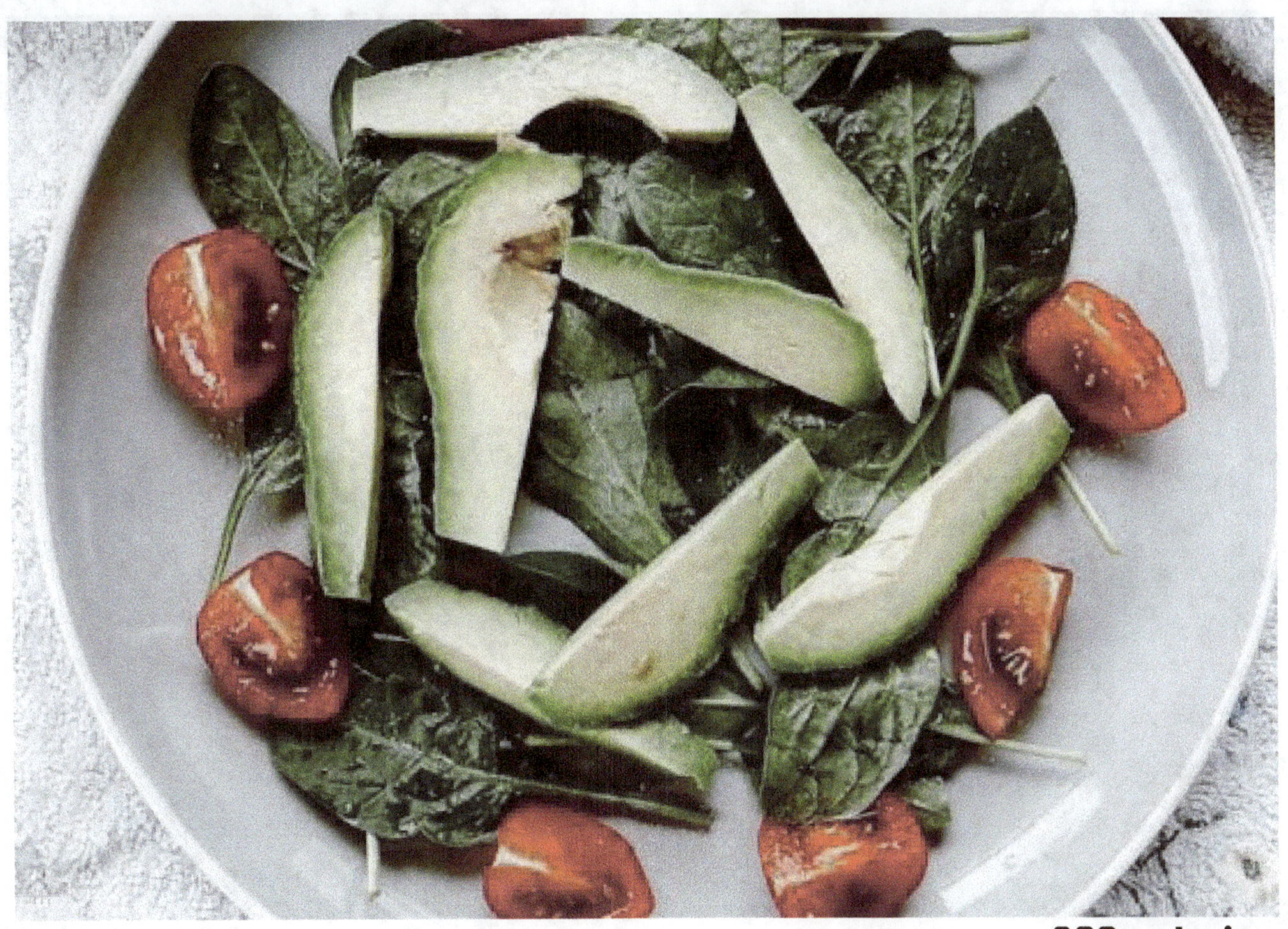

300 calories

What You'll Need:

- 2 cups kale, chopped
- ½ avocado, sliced
- ¼ cup cherry tomatoes, halved
- 2 tbsp lemon juice
- 1 tbsp olive oil

Directions:

- Massage kale with lemon juice and olive oil until tender.
- Top with avocado and cherry tomatoes.
- Toss and serve.

CHICKPEA AND TOMATO SALAD

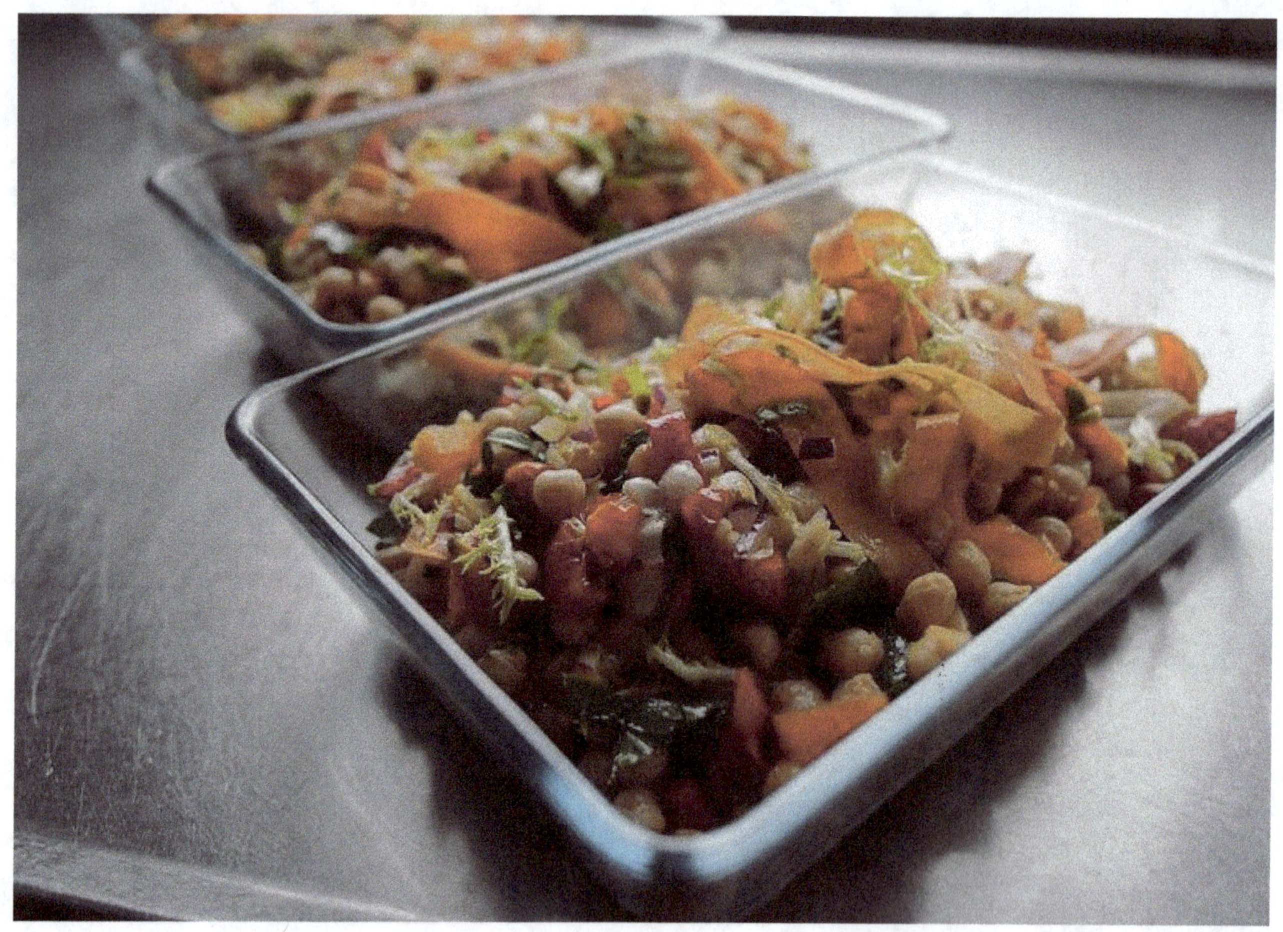

What You'll Need:

- 1 cup canned chickpeas, drained and rinsed
- 1 cup cherry tomatoes, halved
- ¼ cup red onion, finely chopped
- 2 tbsp olive oil
- 1 tbsp lemon juice
- ¼ cup fresh parsley, chopped

Directions:

- Combine chickpeas, cherry tomatoes, and red onion in a bowl.
- Drizzle with olive oil and lemon juice.
- Sprinkle with parsley and toss to mix.

MIXED GREENS WITH BALSAMIC VINAIGRETTE

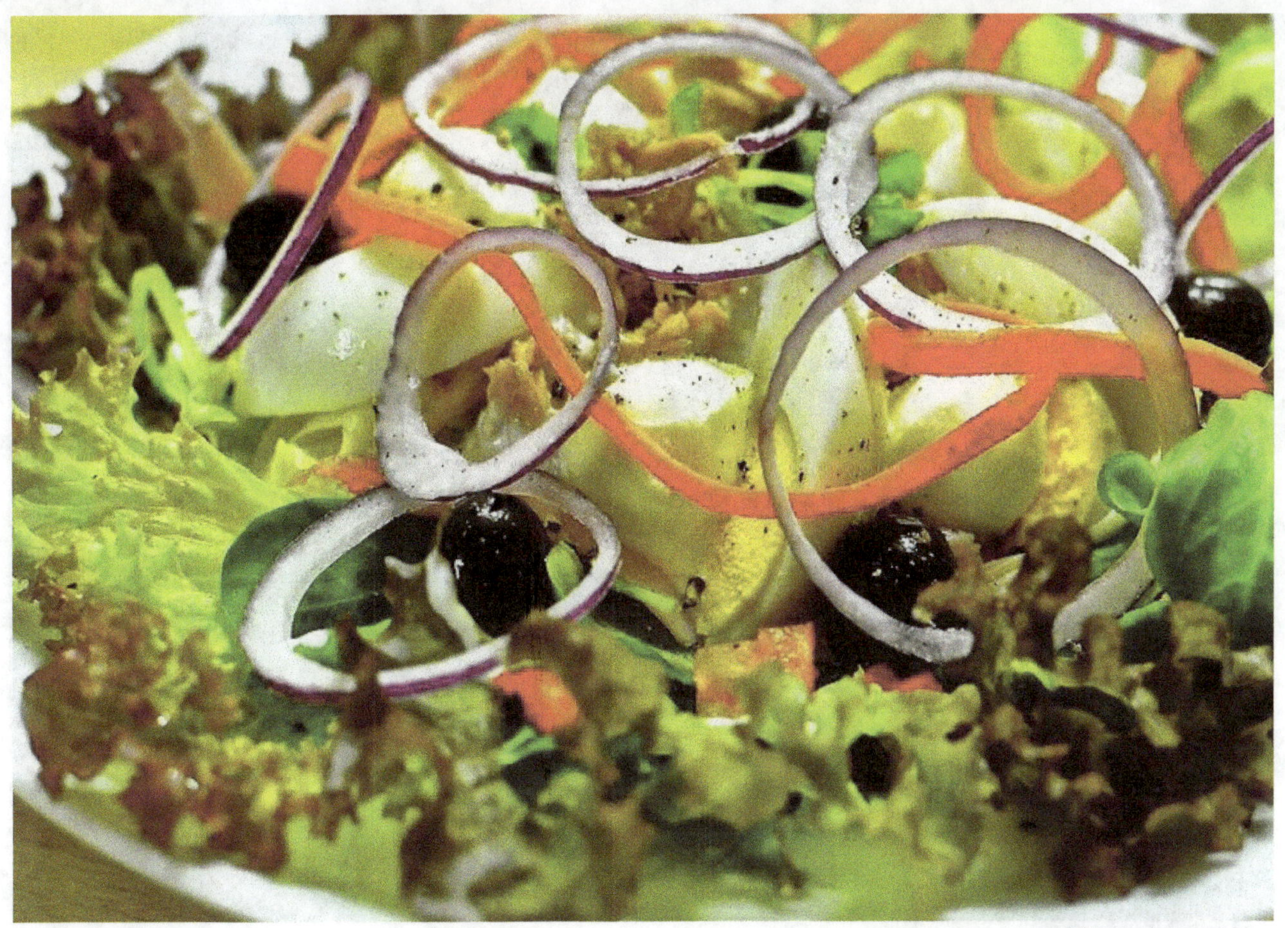

150 calories

What You'll Need:

- 2 cups mixed greens
- 2 tbsp balsamic vinaigrette

Directions:

- Place mixed greens in a bowl.
- Drizzle with balsamic vinaigrette.
- Toss and serve.

ROASTED BEET SALAD

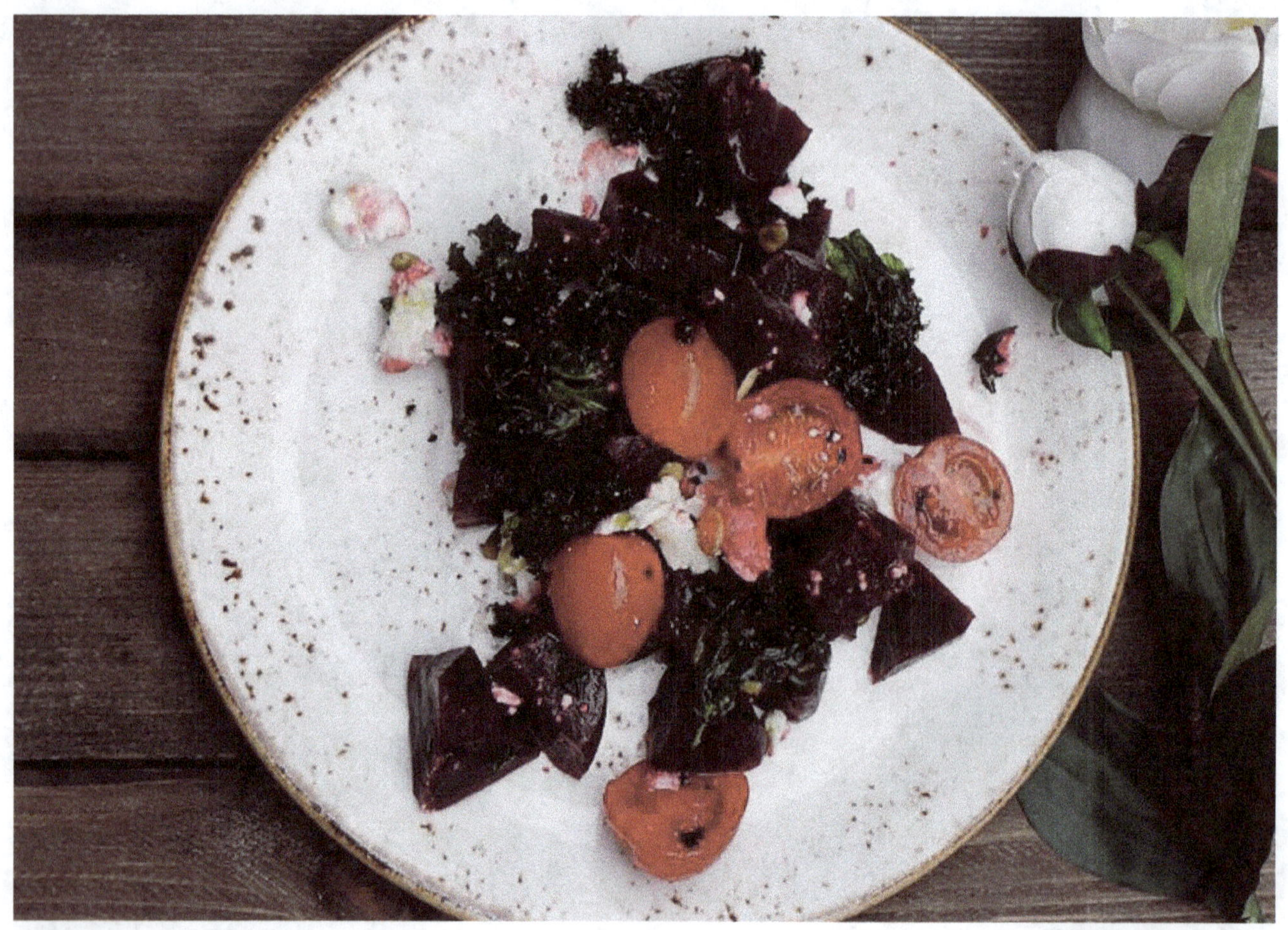

200 calories

What You'll Need:

- 1 cup roasted beets, diced
- 2 cups arugula
- ¼ cup goat cheese, crumbled
- 2 tbsp olive oil
- 1 tbsp balsamic vinegar

Directions:

- Combine roasted beets and arugula in a bowl.
- Top with goat cheese.
- Drizzle with olive oil and balsamic vinegar, then toss.

ASIAN SLAW

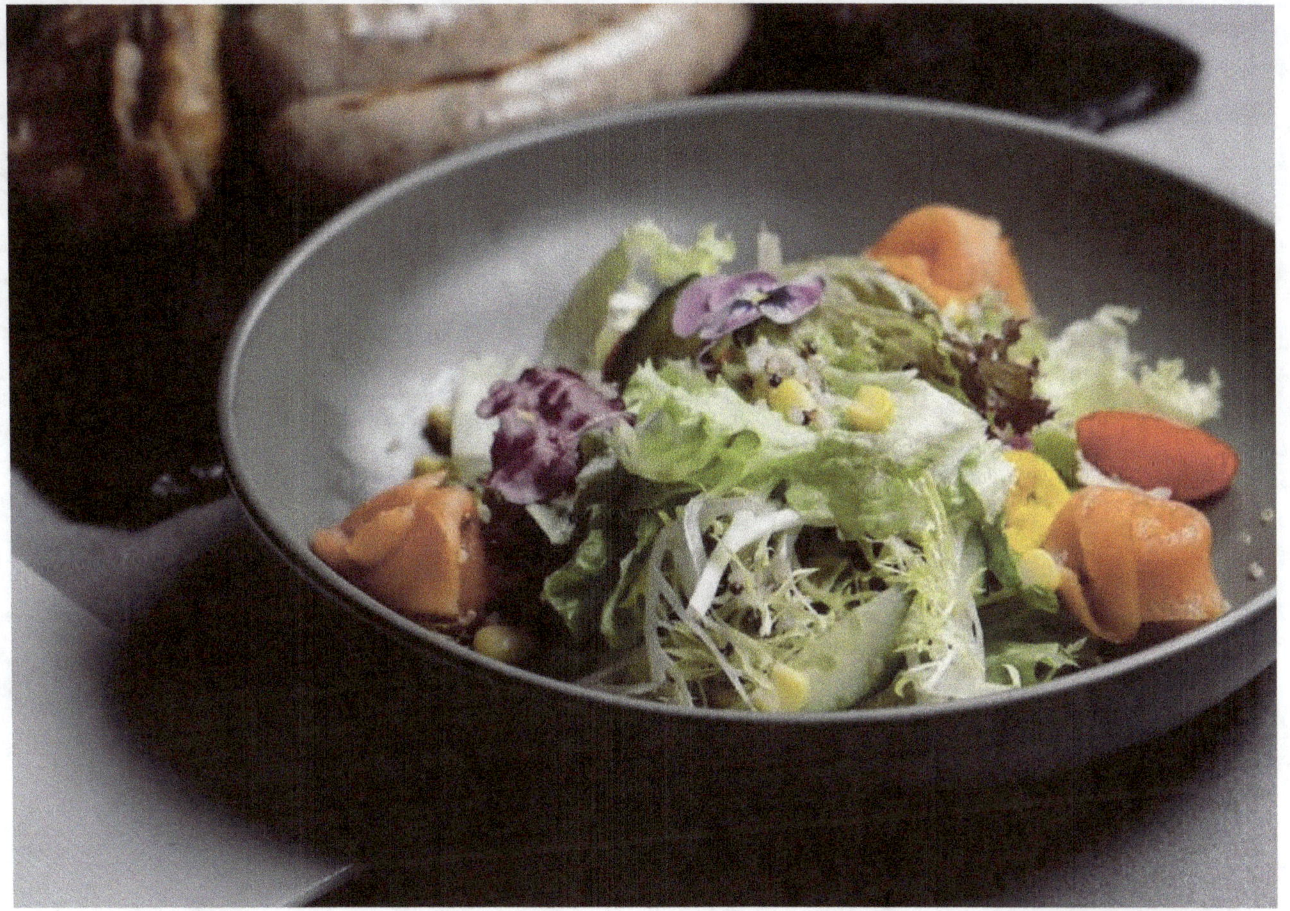

180 calories

<u>**What You'll Need:**</u>

- 2 cups shredded cabbage
- ½ cup shredded carrots
- ¼ cup sliced green onions
- 2 tbsp sesame dressing

<u>**Directions:**</u>

- Combine shredded cabbage, carrots, and green onions in a bowl.
- Drizzle with sesame dressing and toss well.

CAPRESE SALAD

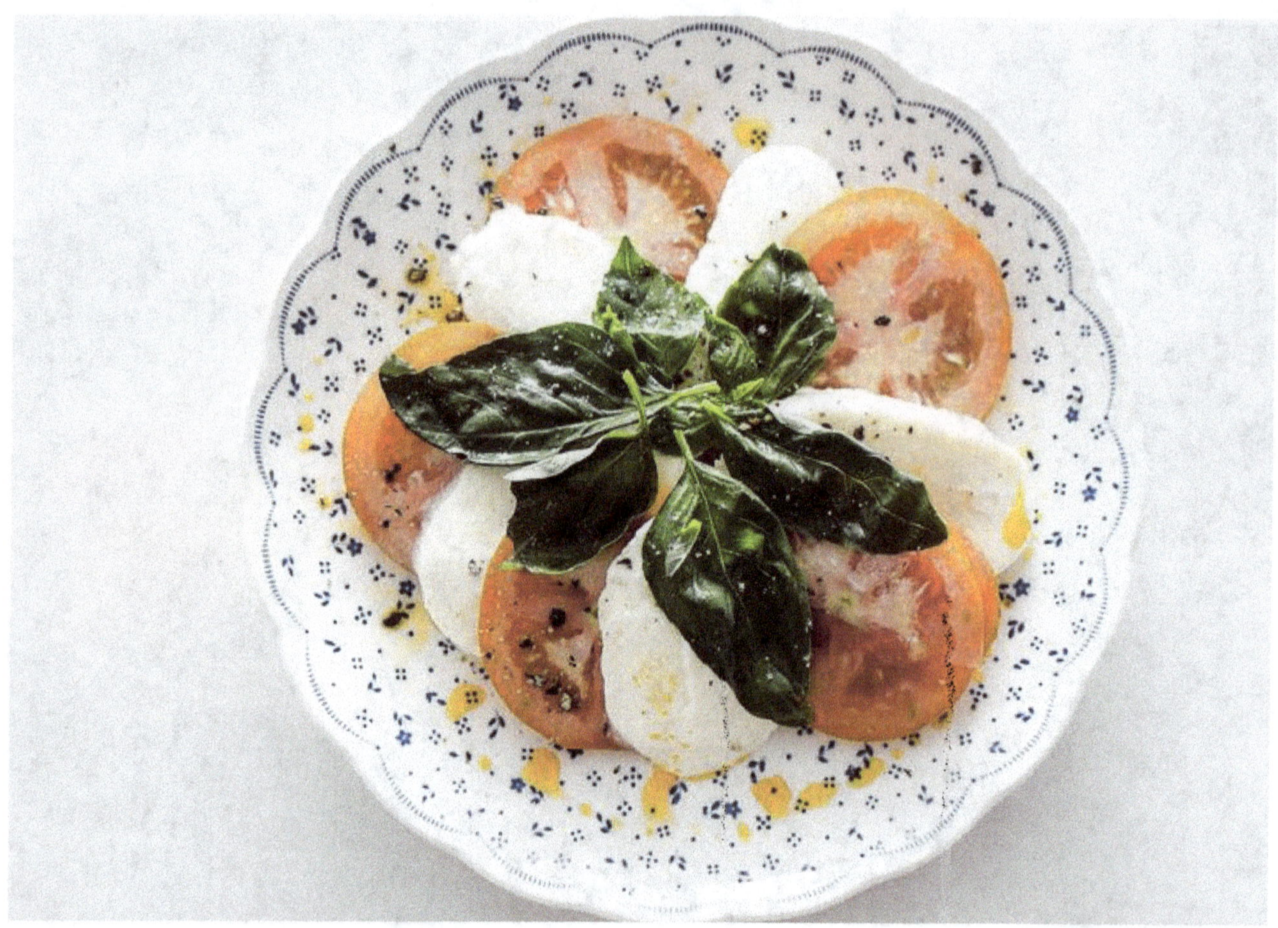

250 calories

<u>**What You'll Need:**</u>

- 1 cup cherry tomatoes, halved
- ¼ cup fresh mozzarella balls
- 2 tbsp fresh basil leaves
- 1 tbsp olive oil
- 1 tbsp balsamic glaze

<u>**Directions:**</u>

- Arrange cherry tomatoes, mozzarella, and basil on a plate.
- Drizzle with olive oil and balsamic glaze.
- Serve immediately.

WRAPS AND SANDWICHES

TURKEY AND AVOCADO WRAP

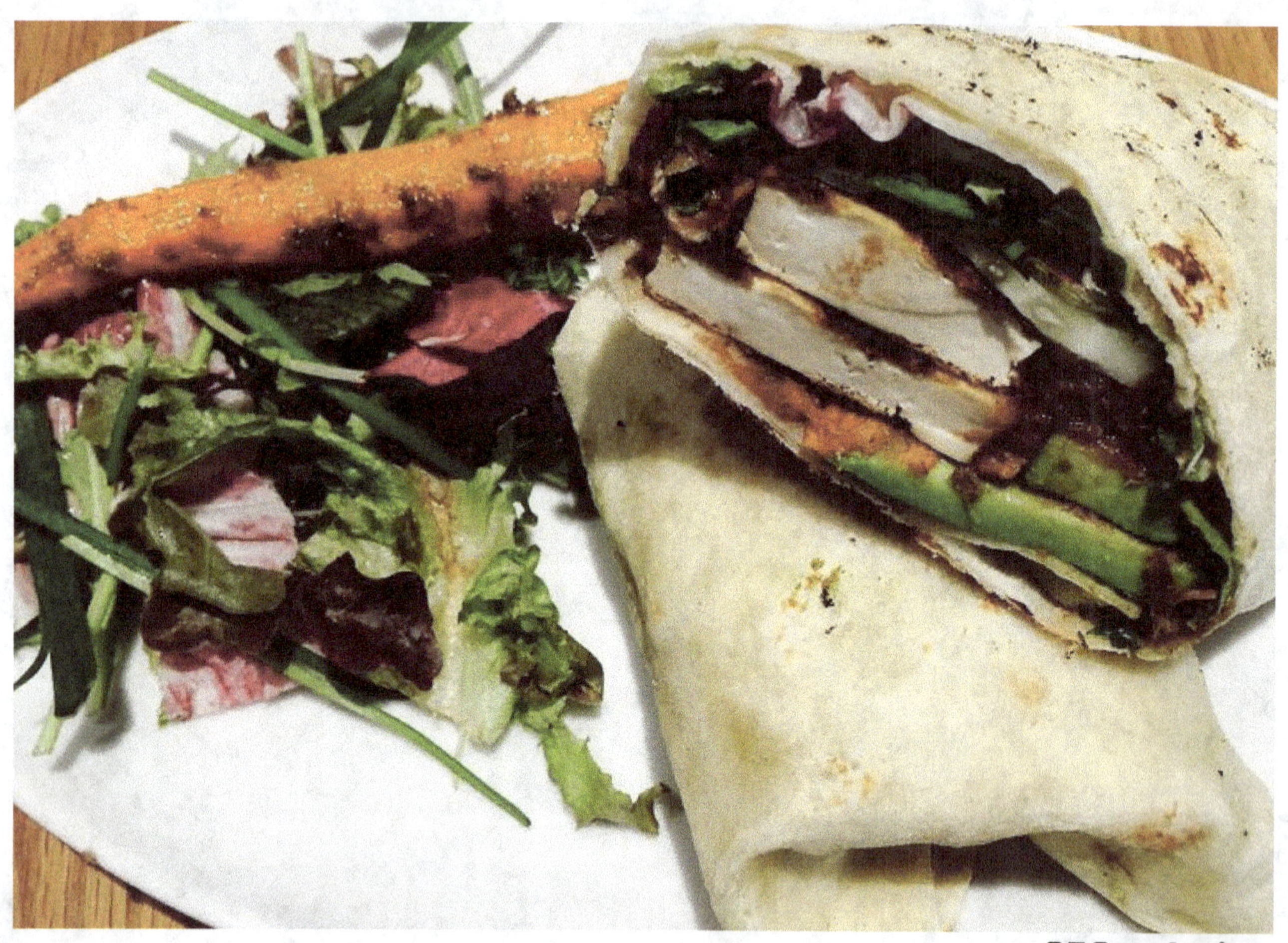

350 calories

What You'll Need:

- 1 whole wheat tortilla
- 3 oz turkey breast
- ¼ avocado, sliced
- 1 cup lettuce, sliced
- 1 tbsp mustard

Directions:

- Layer turkey, avocado, and lettuce on the tortilla.
- Spread mustard.
- Roll up the tortilla to enclose the filling.

CHICKEN CAESAR WRAP

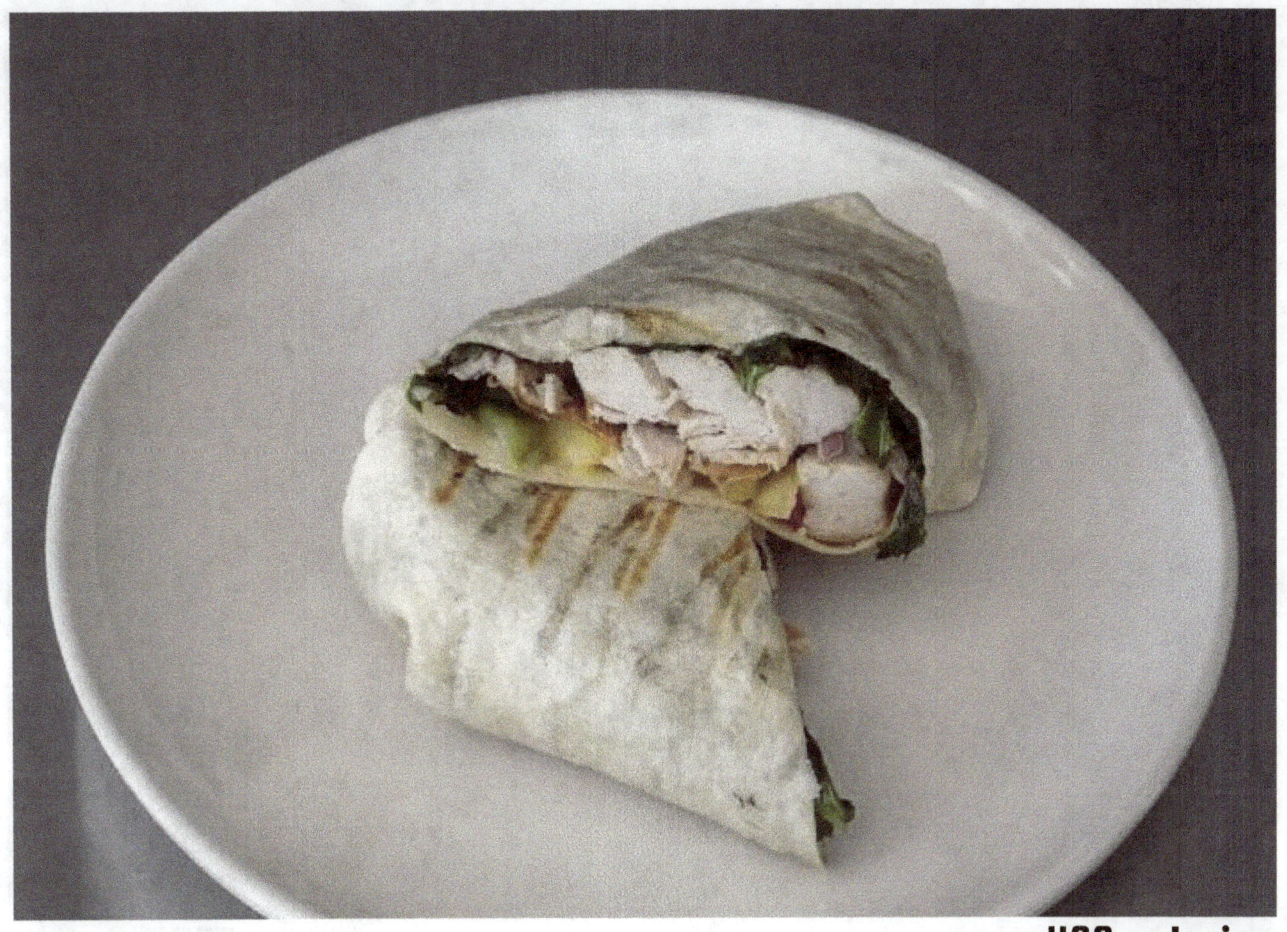

400 calories

What You'll Need:

- 1 whole wheat tortilla
- 3 oz grilled chicken
- 2 tbsp Caesar dressing
- 1 cup romaine lettuce
- ¼ cup Parmesan cheese

Directions:

- Toss grilled chicken with Caesar dressing.
- Layer on the tortilla with romaine lettuce and Parmesan cheese.
- Roll up the tortilla.

VEGGIE HUMMUS WRAP

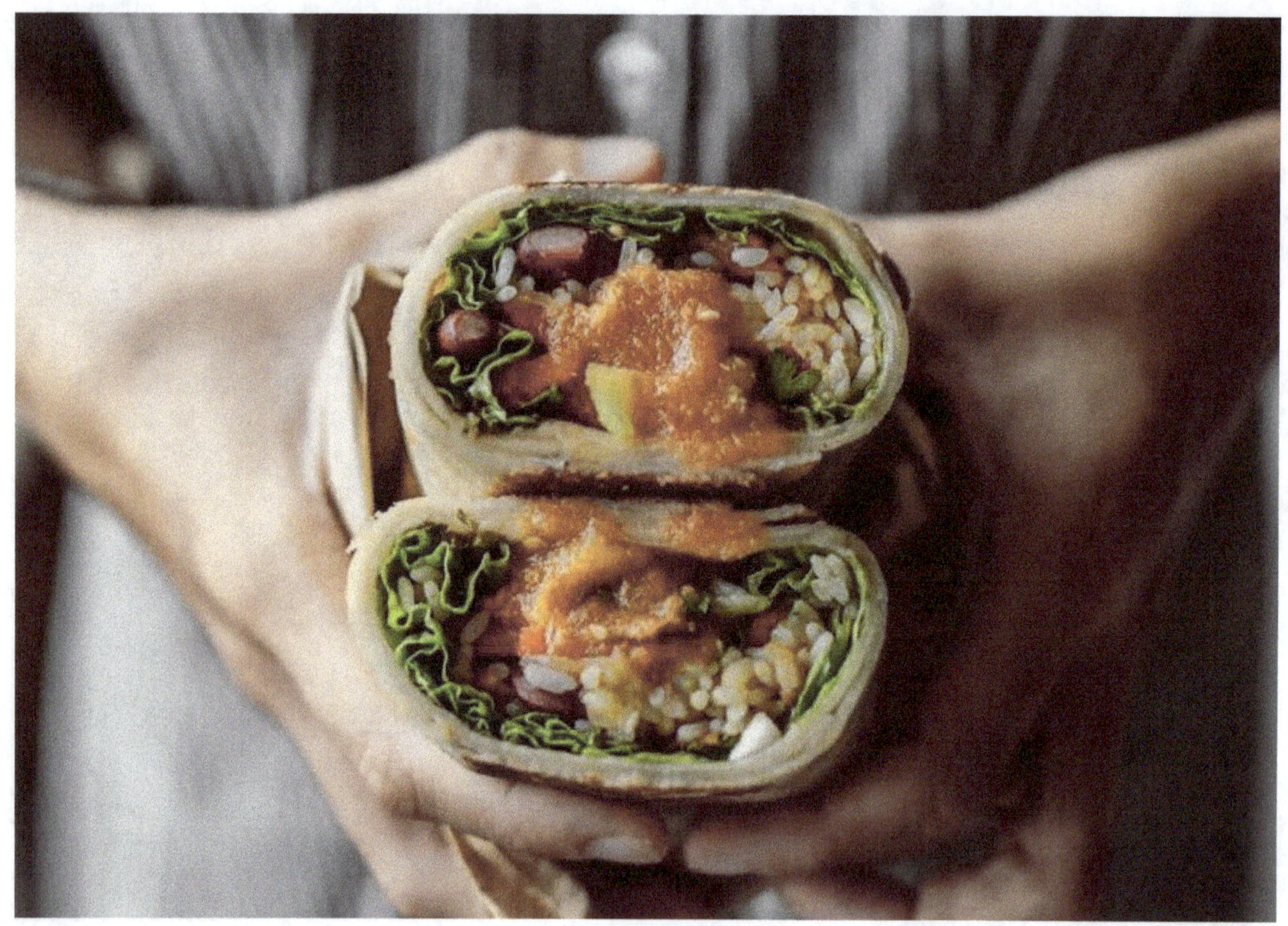

300 calories

What You'll Need:

- 1 whole wheat tortilla
- ¼ cup hummus
- 1 cup mixed vegetables (e.g., bell peppers, cucumbers, carrots)
- 1 cup spinach

Directions:

- Spread hummus on the tortilla.
- Layer with mixed vegetables and spinach.
- Roll up the tortilla.

TUNA SALAD SANDWICH

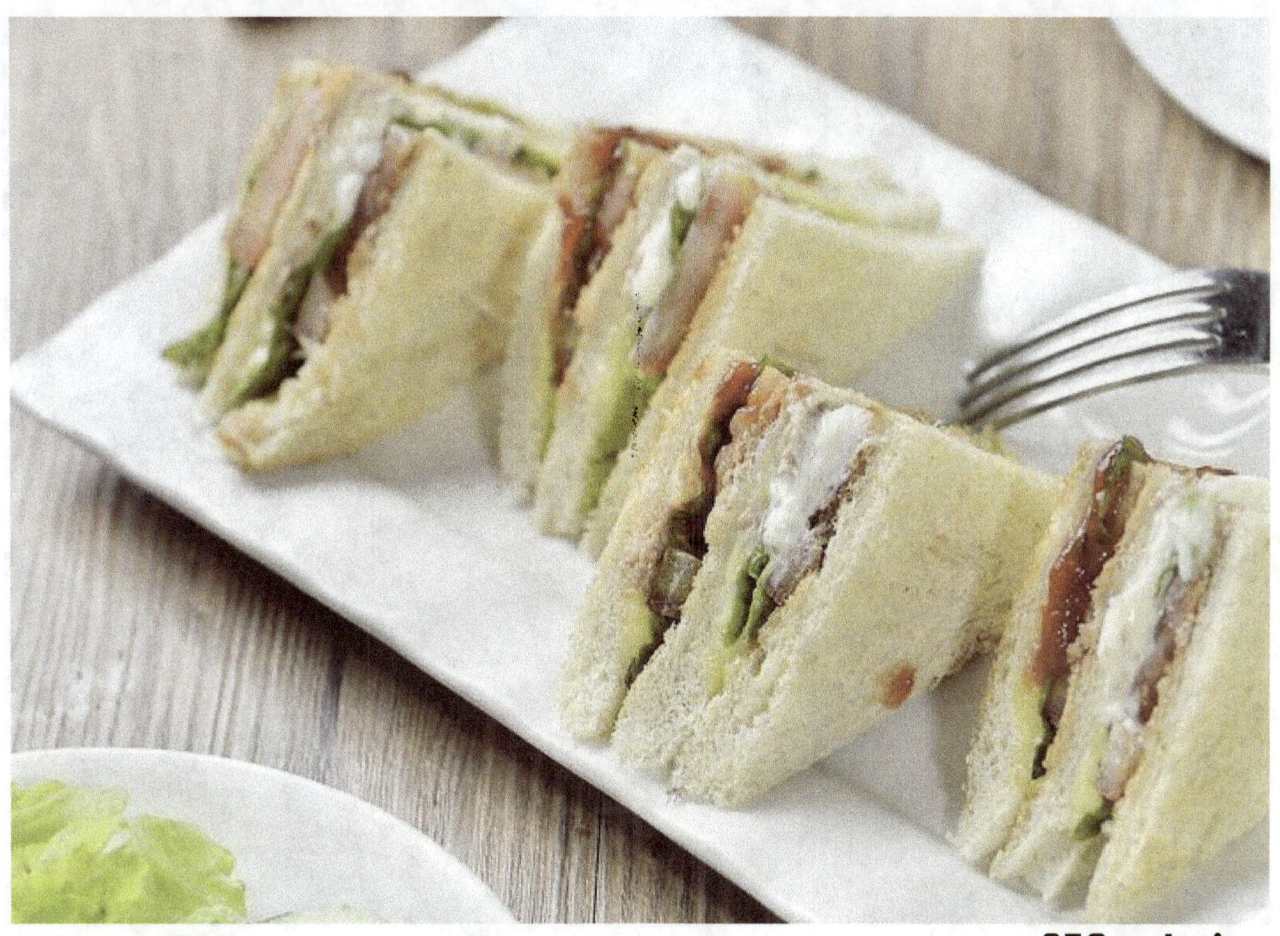

350 calories

What You'll Need:

- 2 slices whole grain bread
- 1 can tuna, drained
- 2 tbsp Greek yogurt
- 1 tbsp mustard
- ¼ cup celery, chopped

Directions:

- Mix tuna with Greek yogurt, mustard, and celery.
- Spread the mixture on one slice of bread.
- Top with the other slice and cut the sandwich in half.

CAPRESE SANDWICH

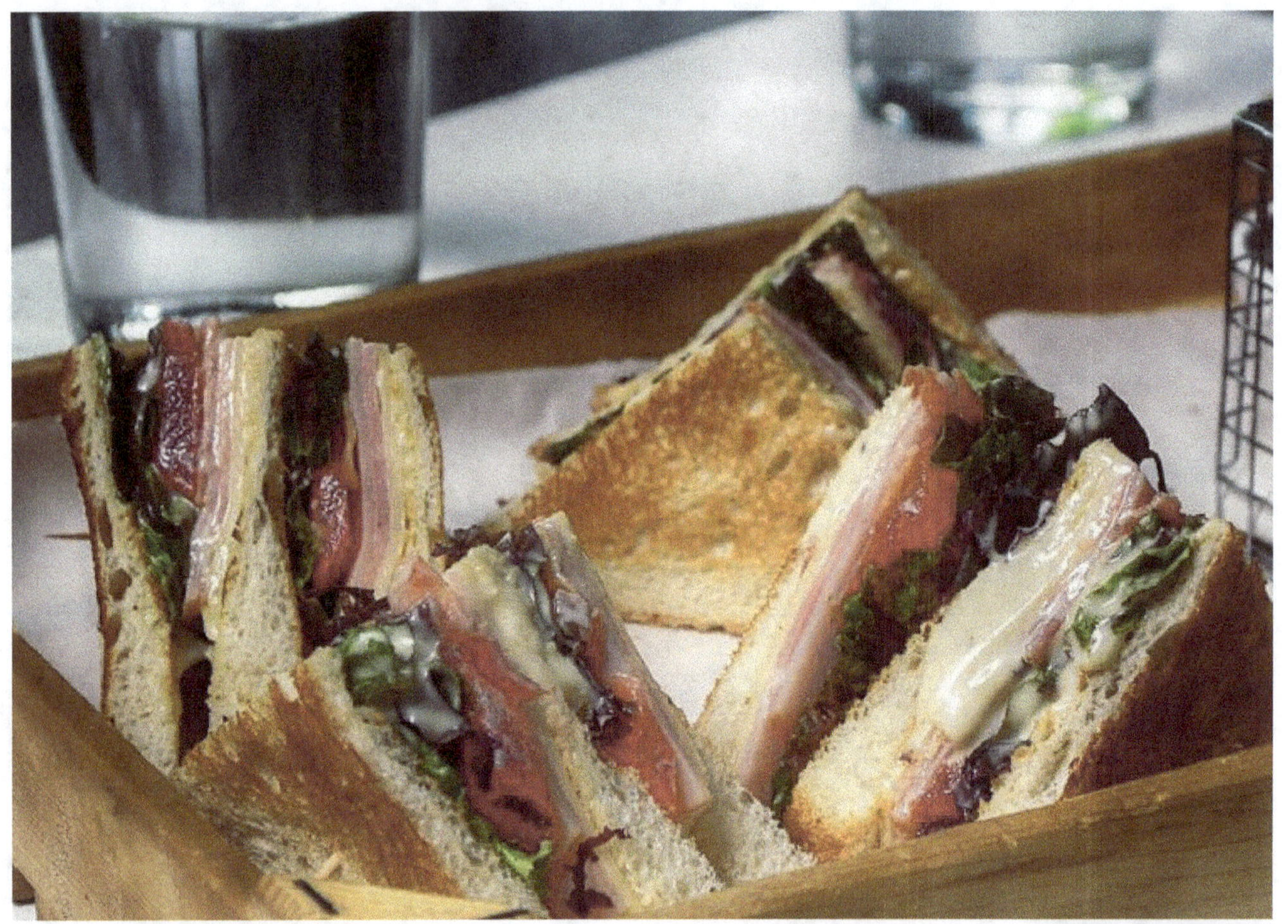

300 calories

What You'll Need:

- 2 slices whole grain bread
- ¼ cup fresh mozzarella
- 2 slices tomato
- 2 leaves basil
- 1 tbsp balsamic glaze

Directions:

- Layer mozzarella, tomato, and basil on one slice of bread.
- Drizzle with balsamic glaze.
- Top with the other slice of bread and press down.

GREEK PITA POCKET

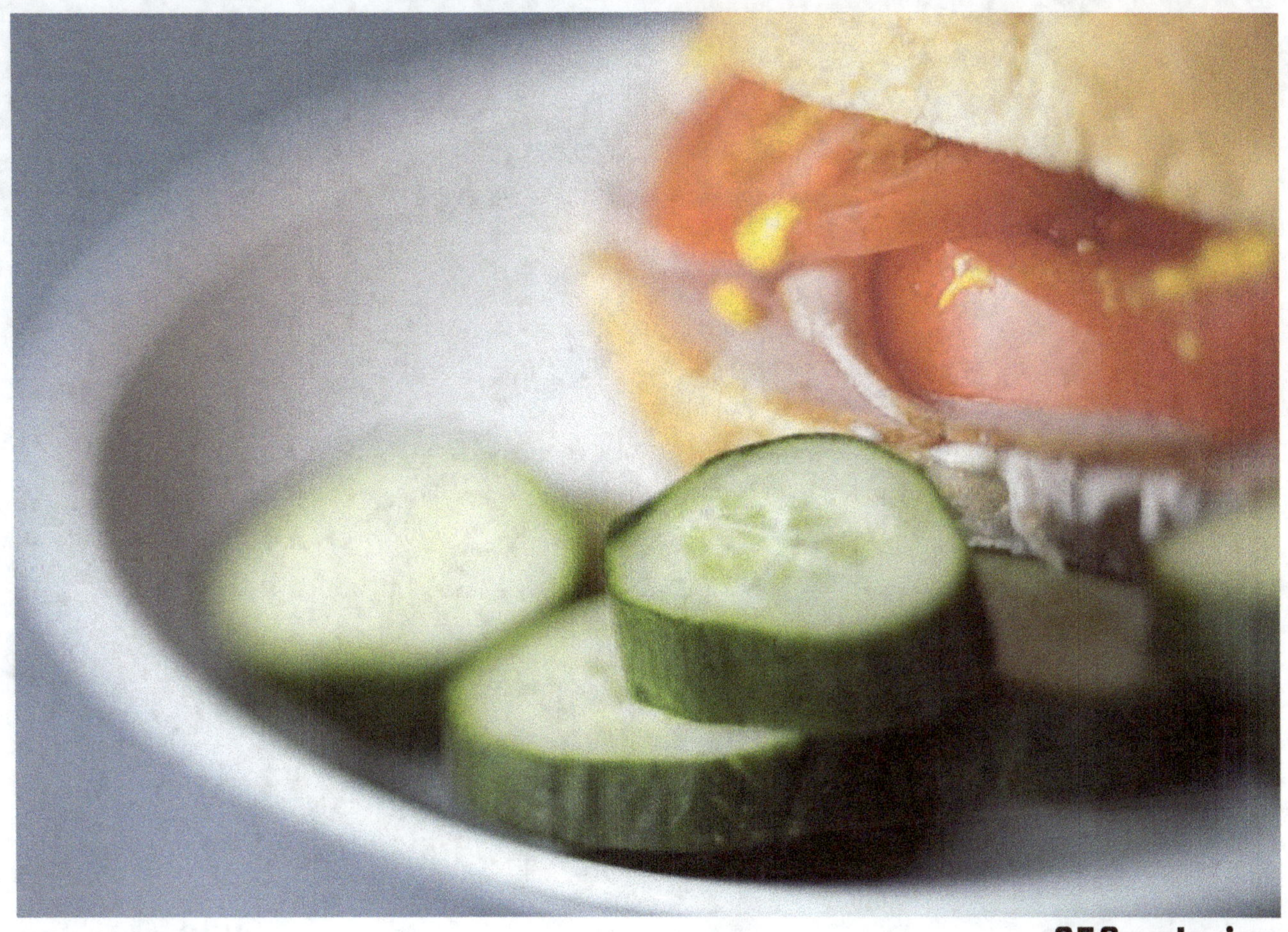

350 calories

What You'll Need:

- 1 whole wheat pita
- ¼ cup feta cheese
- ½ cup cucumber, diced
- ½ cup tomatoes, diced
- 2 tbsp tzatziki sauce

Directions:

- Cut pita in half and gently open to create pockets.
- Stuff with feta cheese, cucumber, and tomatoes.
- Add tzatziki sauce before serving.

BUFFALO CHICKEN WRAP

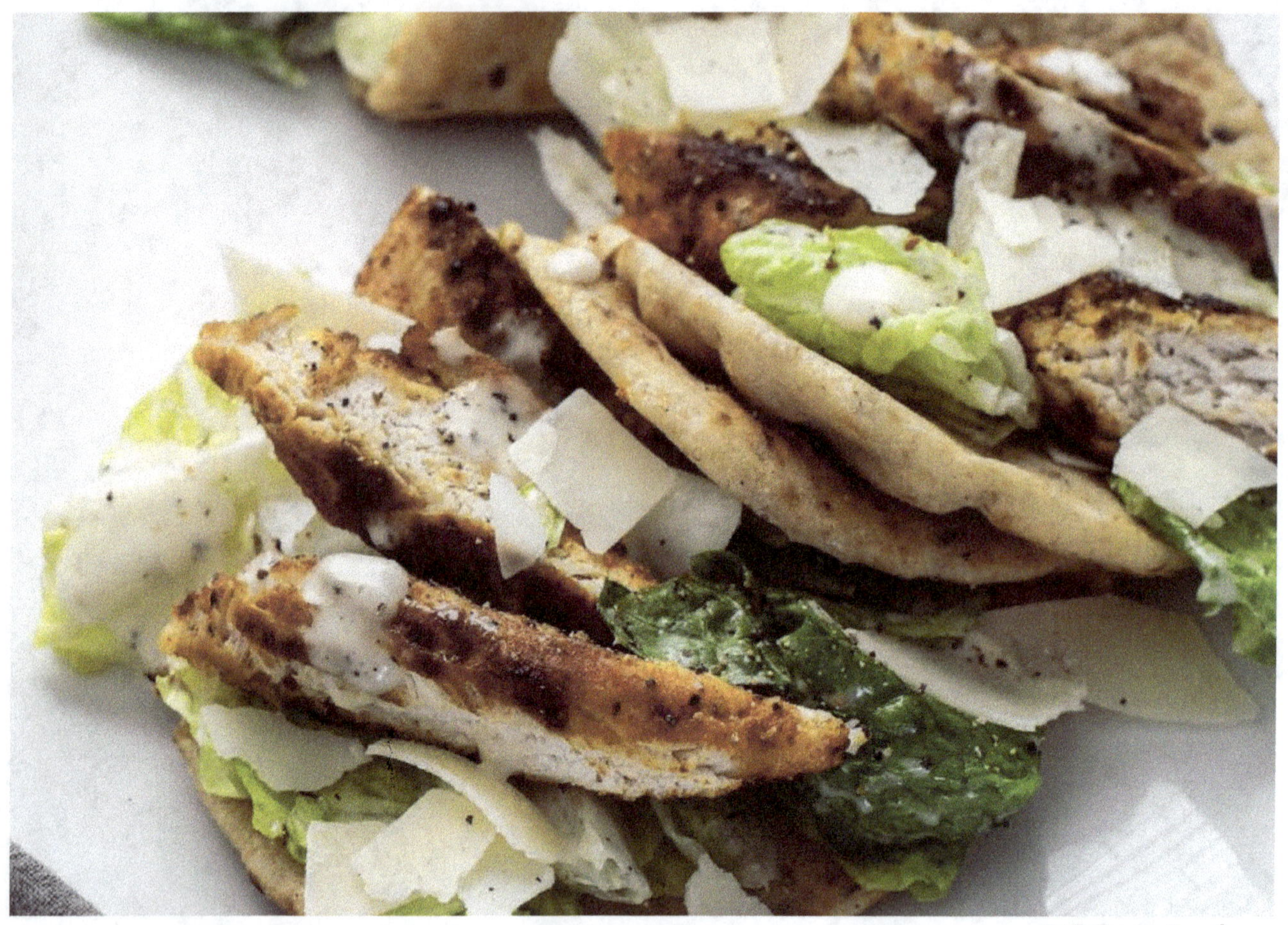

400 calories

What You'll Need:

- 1 whole wheat tortilla
- 3 oz shredded chicken
- 2 tbsp buffalo sauce
- 1 cup lettuce
- 2 tbsp ranch dressing

Directions:

- Toss shredded chicken with buffalo sauce.
- Layer on the tortilla with lettuce and ranch dressing.
- Roll up the tortilla.

EGG SALAD SANDWICH

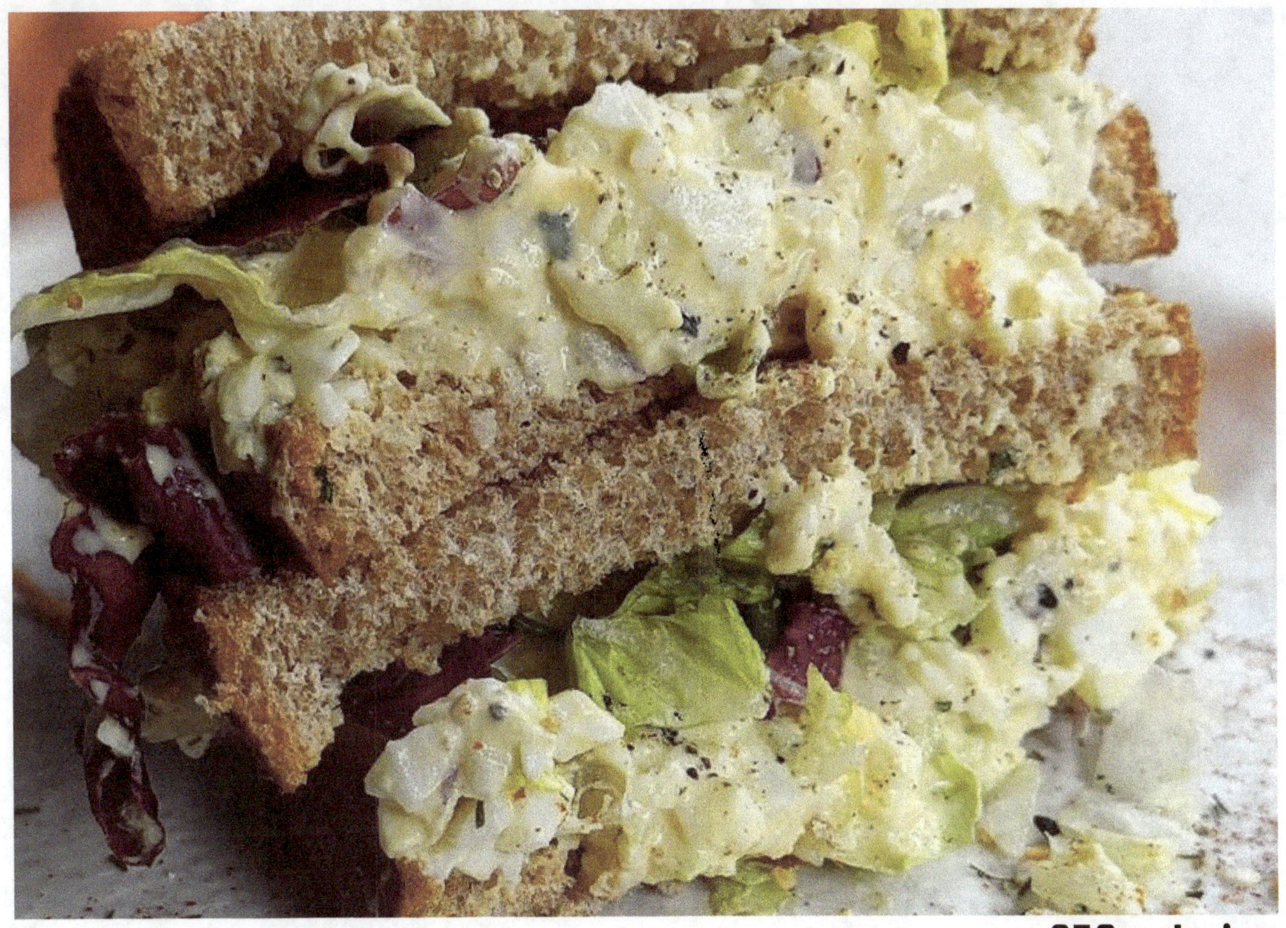

350 calories

What You'll Need:

- 2 slices whole grain bread
- 2 hard-boiled eggs, chopped
- 2 tbsp Greek yogurt
- 1 tbsp mustard
- ¼ cup celery, chopped

Directions:

- Mash chopped eggs and mix with Greek yogurt, mustard, and celery.
- Spread the mixture on one slice of bread.
- Top with the other slice and cut the sandwich in half.

BLACK BEAN AND CORN WRAP

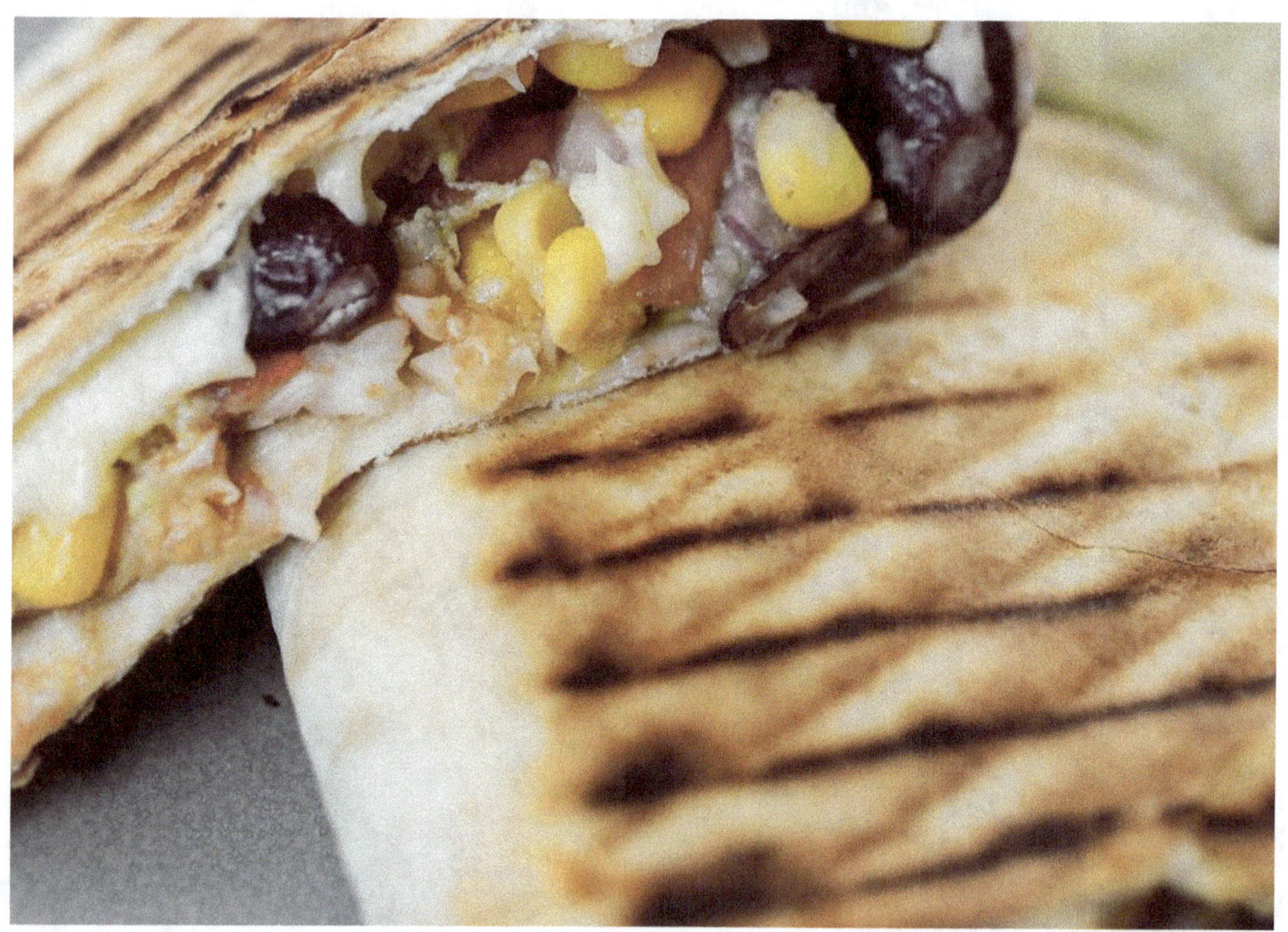

300 calories

What You'll Need:

- 1 whole wheat tortilla
- ½ cup black beans
- ½ cup corn
- ¼ cup shredded cheese
- 2 tbsp salsa

Directions:

- Layer black beans, corn, and cheese on the tortilla.
- Top with salsa.
- Roll up the tortilla.

TURKEY AND SWISS SANDWICH

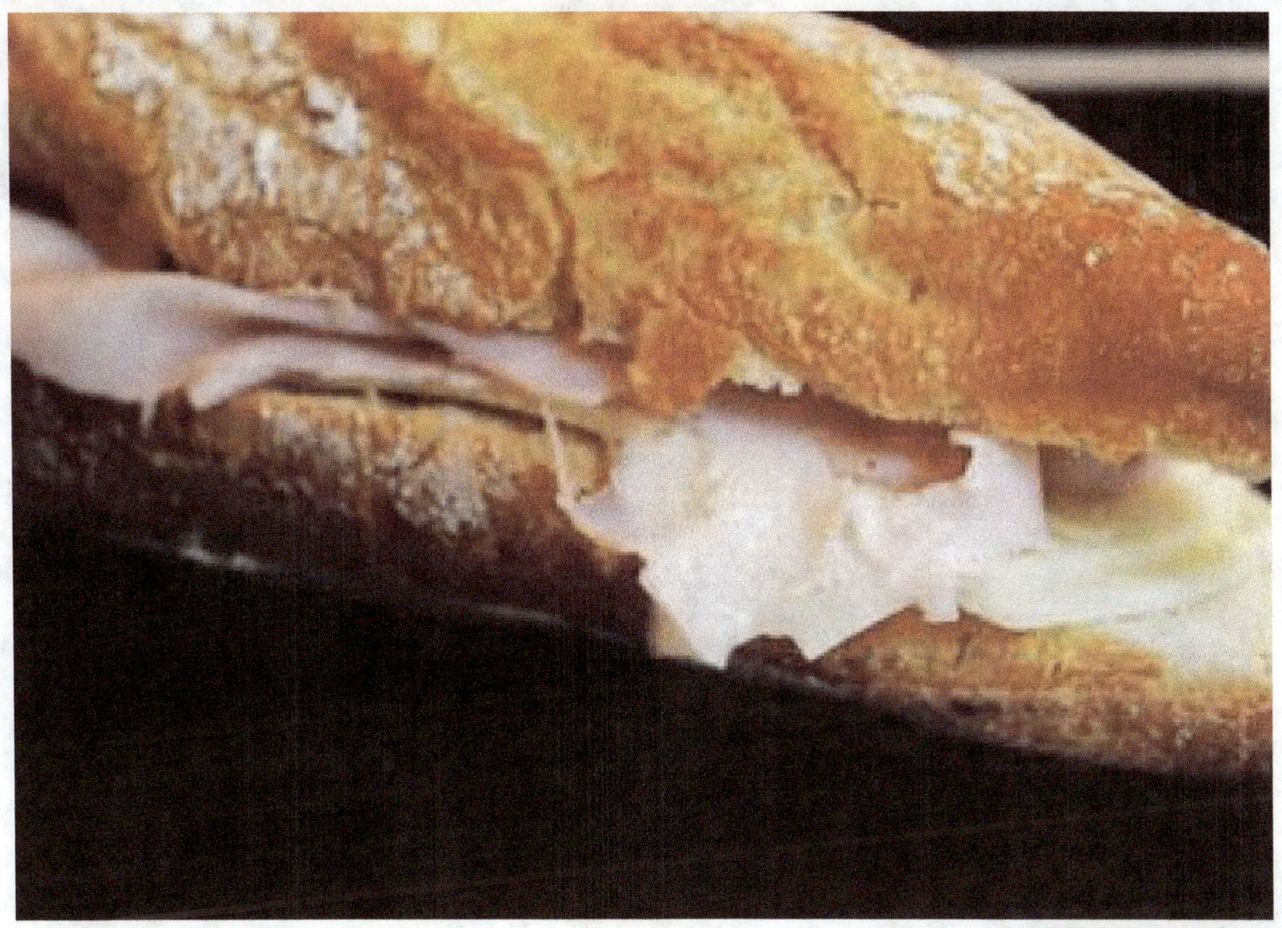

350 calories

What You'll Need:

- 2 slices whole grain bread
- 3 oz turkey breast
- 1 slice Swiss cheese
- 1 tbsp mustard
- 1 cup lettuce

Directions:

- Layer turkey, Swiss cheese, and lettuce on one slice of bread.
- Spread mustard on the other slice.
- Assemble the sandwich and cut it in half.

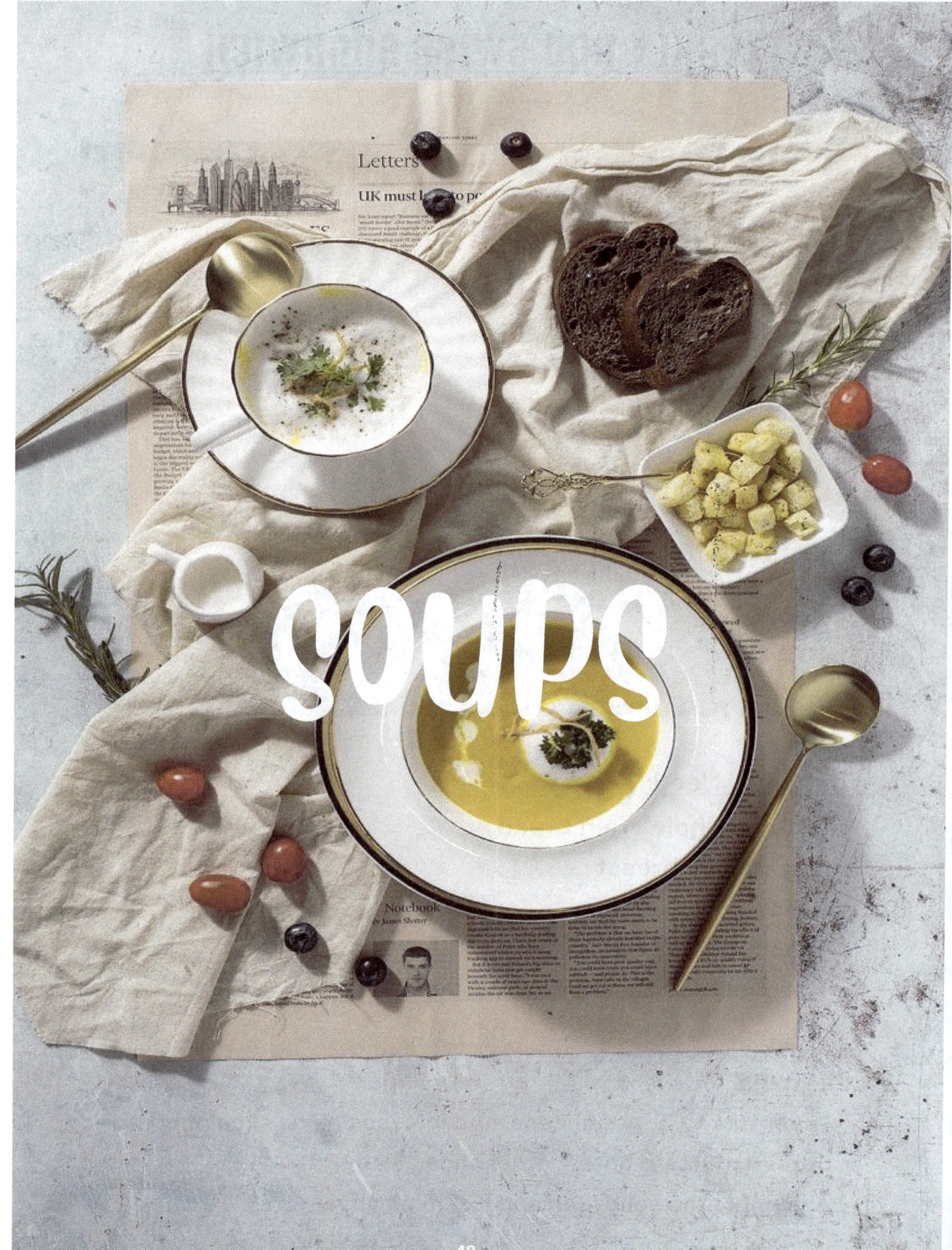
SOUPS

TOMATO BASIL SOUP

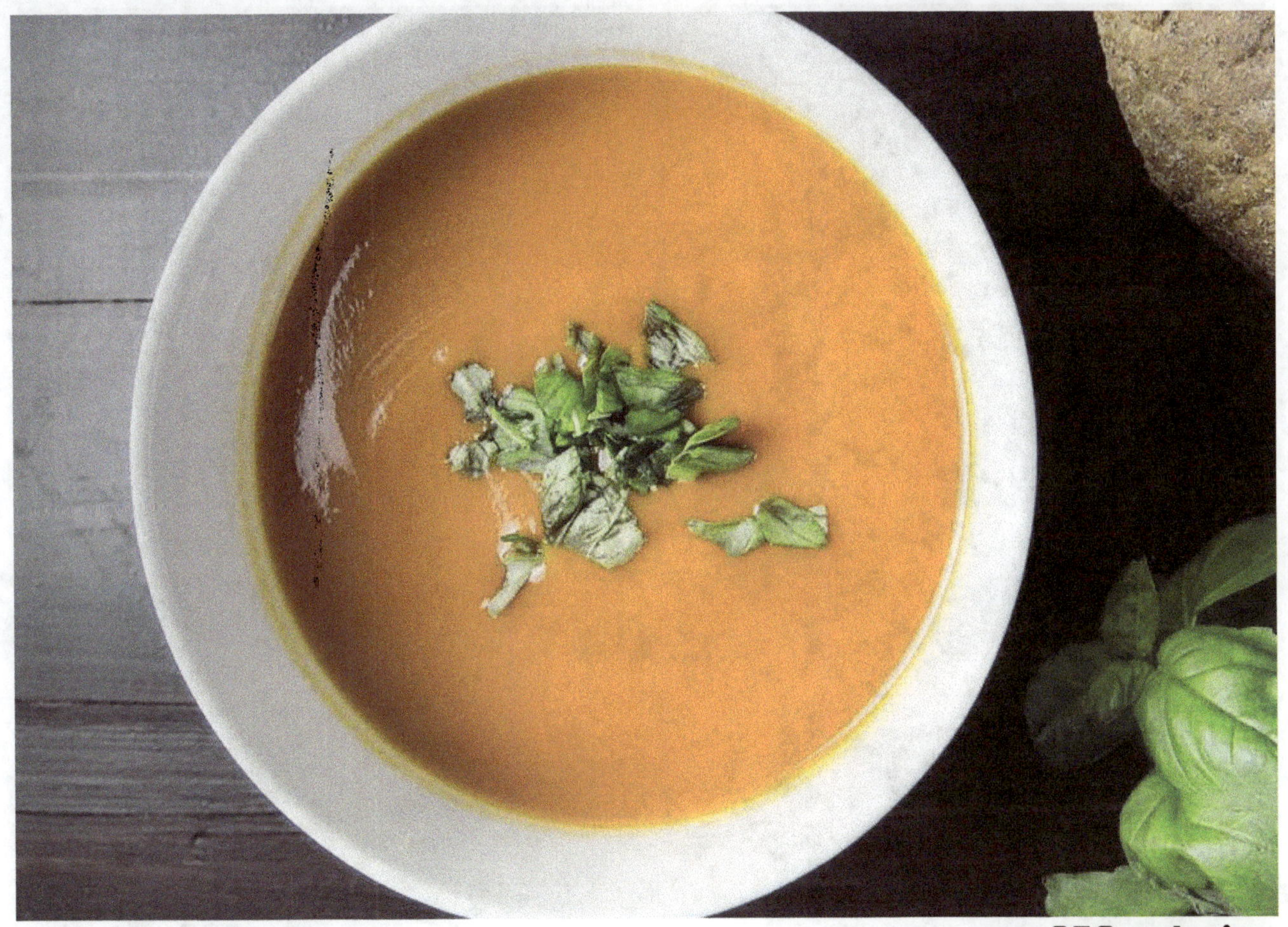

What You'll Need:

- 1 cup tomatoes, chopped
- ¼ cup fresh basil leaves
- 1 cup vegetable broth
- 1 tbsp olive oil

Directions:

- Sauté basil in olive oil until fragrant.
- Add tomatoes and vegetable broth.
- Simmer until tomatoes are soft.
- Blend until smooth and serve.

LENTIL SOUP

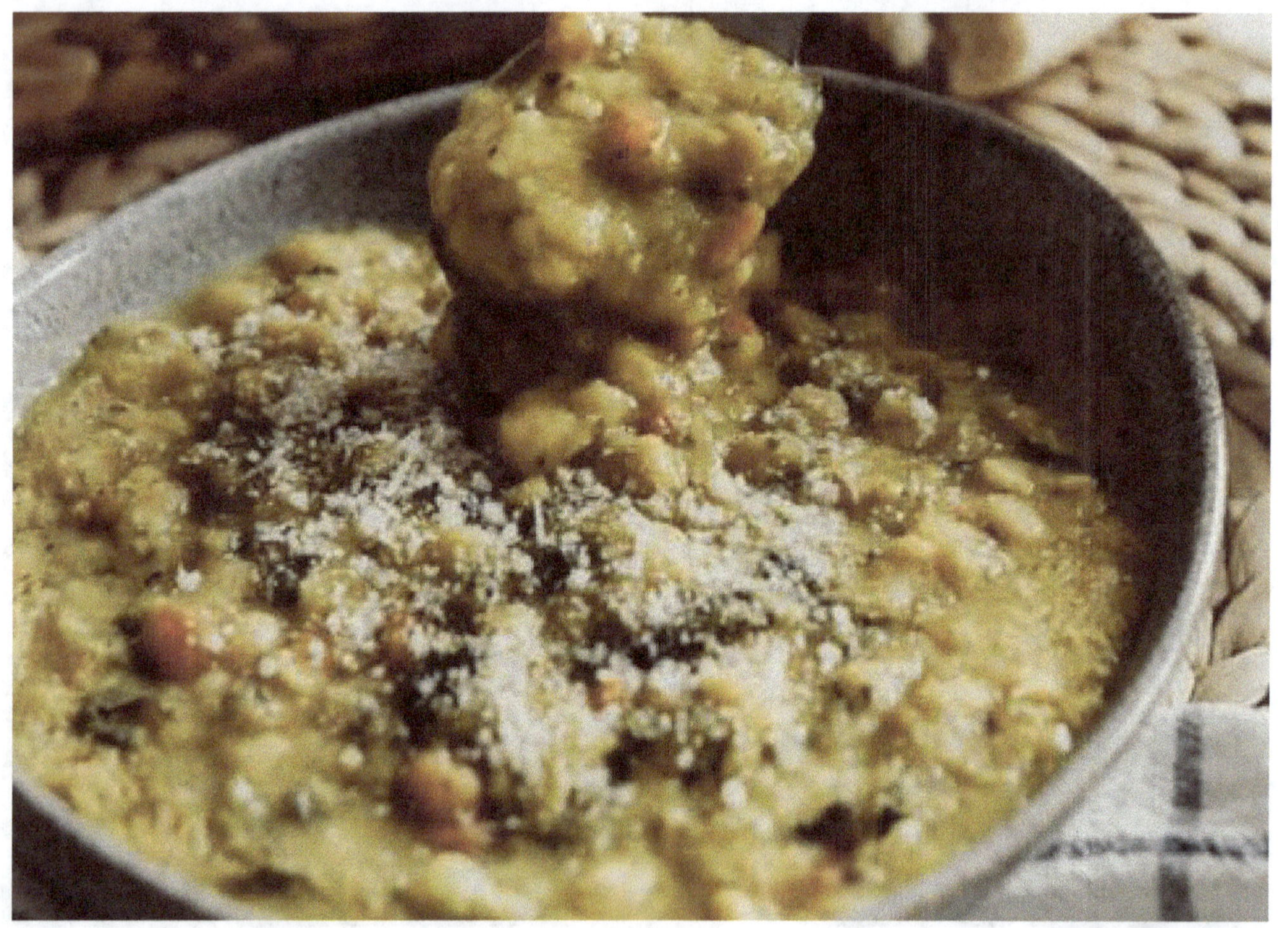

300 calories

What You'll Need:

- 1 cup lentils
- 1 cup carrots, diced
- 1 cup celery, diced
- 1 cup vegetable broth
- 1 tsp cumin

Directions:

- Sauté carrots and celery in a pot until softened.
- Add lentils, vegetable broth, and cumin.
- Simmer until lentils are tender.
- Season to taste and serve.

BUTTERNUT SQUASH SOUP

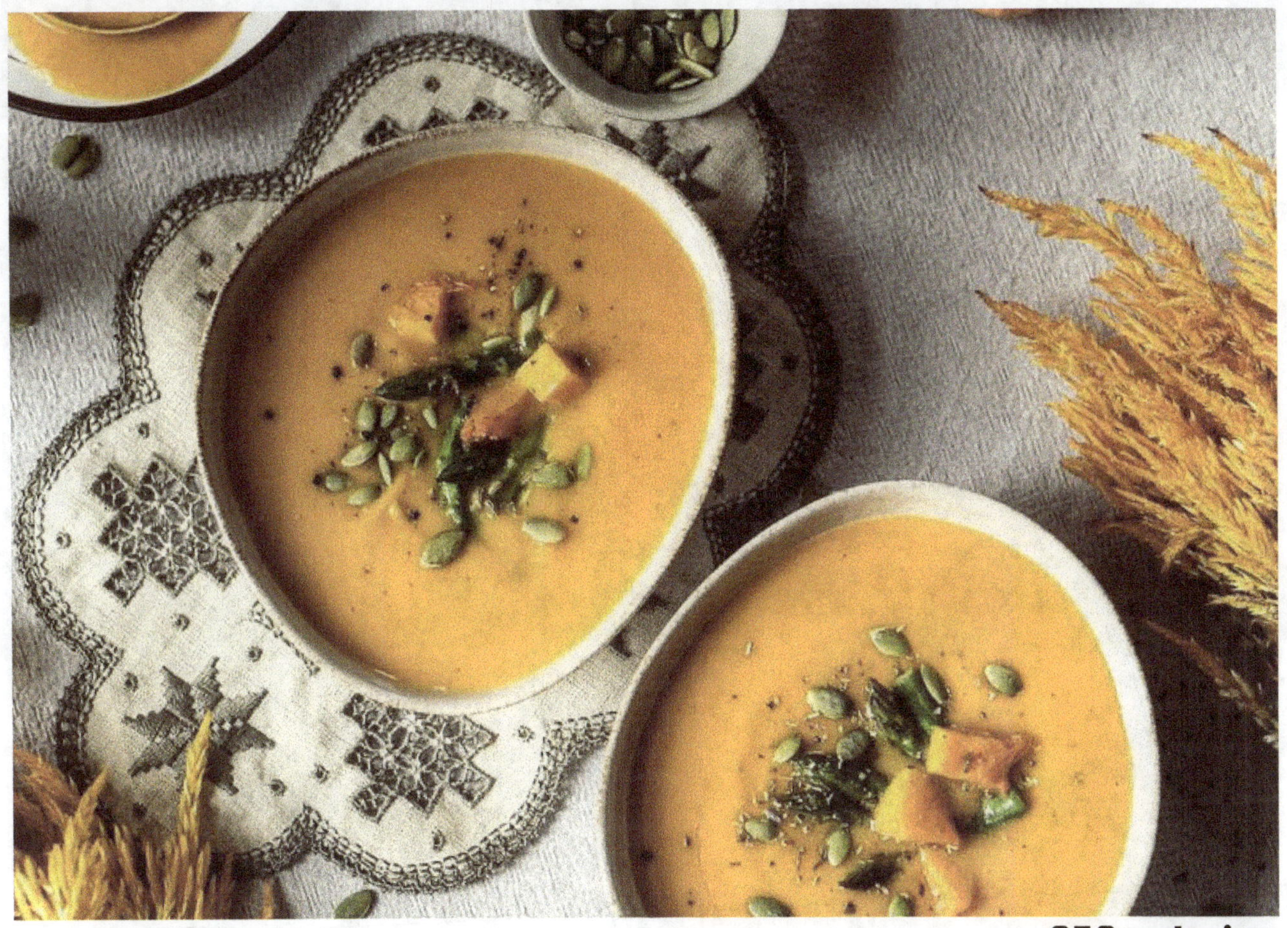

250 calories

What You'll Need:

- 2 cups butternut squash, peeled and diced
- 1 cup vegetable broth
- 1 onion, chopped
- 1 tsp ginger
- 1 tbsp olive oil

Directions:

- Sauté onion and ginger in olive oil until fragrant.
- Add butternut squash and vegetable broth.
- Simmer until squash is tender.
- Blend until smooth and season to taste.

CHICKEN AND VEGETABLE SOUP

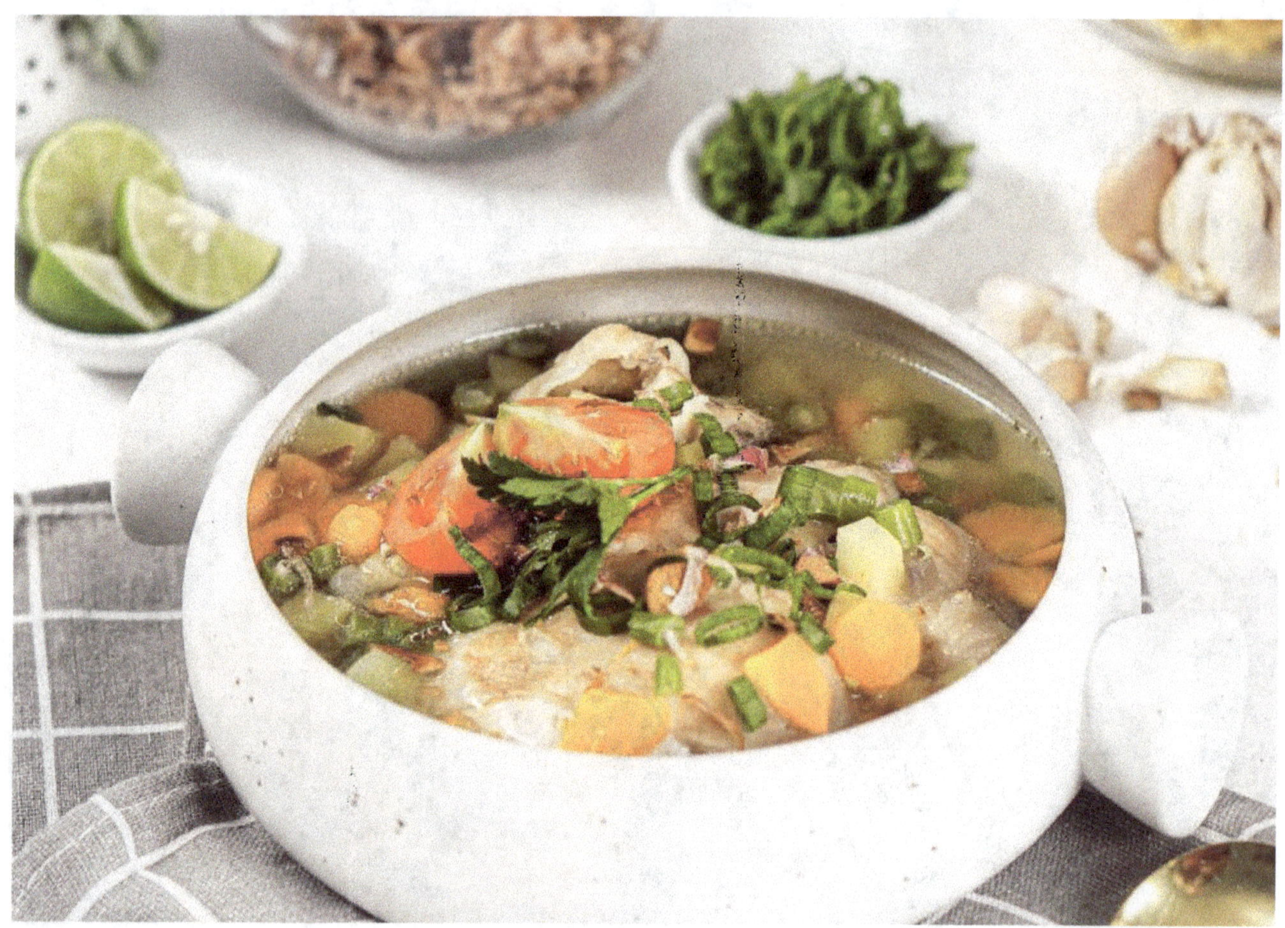

300 calories

What You'll Need:

- 1 cup cooked chicken breast, diced
- 1 cup mixed vegetables (carrots, peas, corn)
- 1 cup chicken broth
- 1 tsp thyme

Directions:

- Combine chicken, vegetables, and chicken broth in a pot.
- Simmer until vegetables are tender.
- Season with thyme and serve.

MINESTRONE SOUP

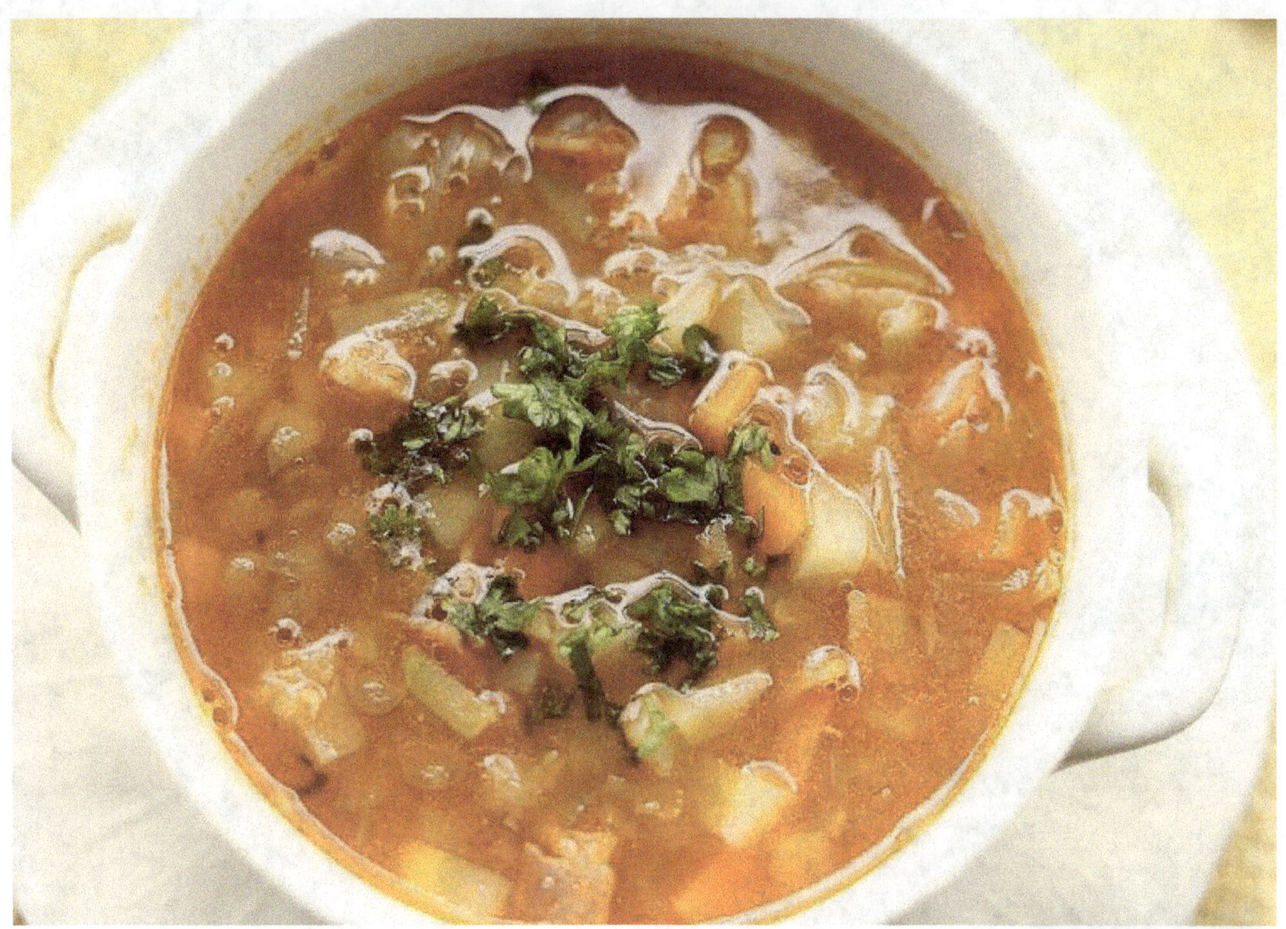

350 calories

What You'll Need:

- 1 cup kidney beans
- 1 cup diced tomatoes
- 1 cup zucchini, diced
- 1 cup vegetable broth
- 1 tsp Italian seasoning

Directions:

- Combine kidney beans, tomatoes, zucchini, and broth in a pot.
- Simmer until vegetables are cooked through.
- Season with Italian seasoning and serve.

SPINACH AND WHITE BEAN SOUP

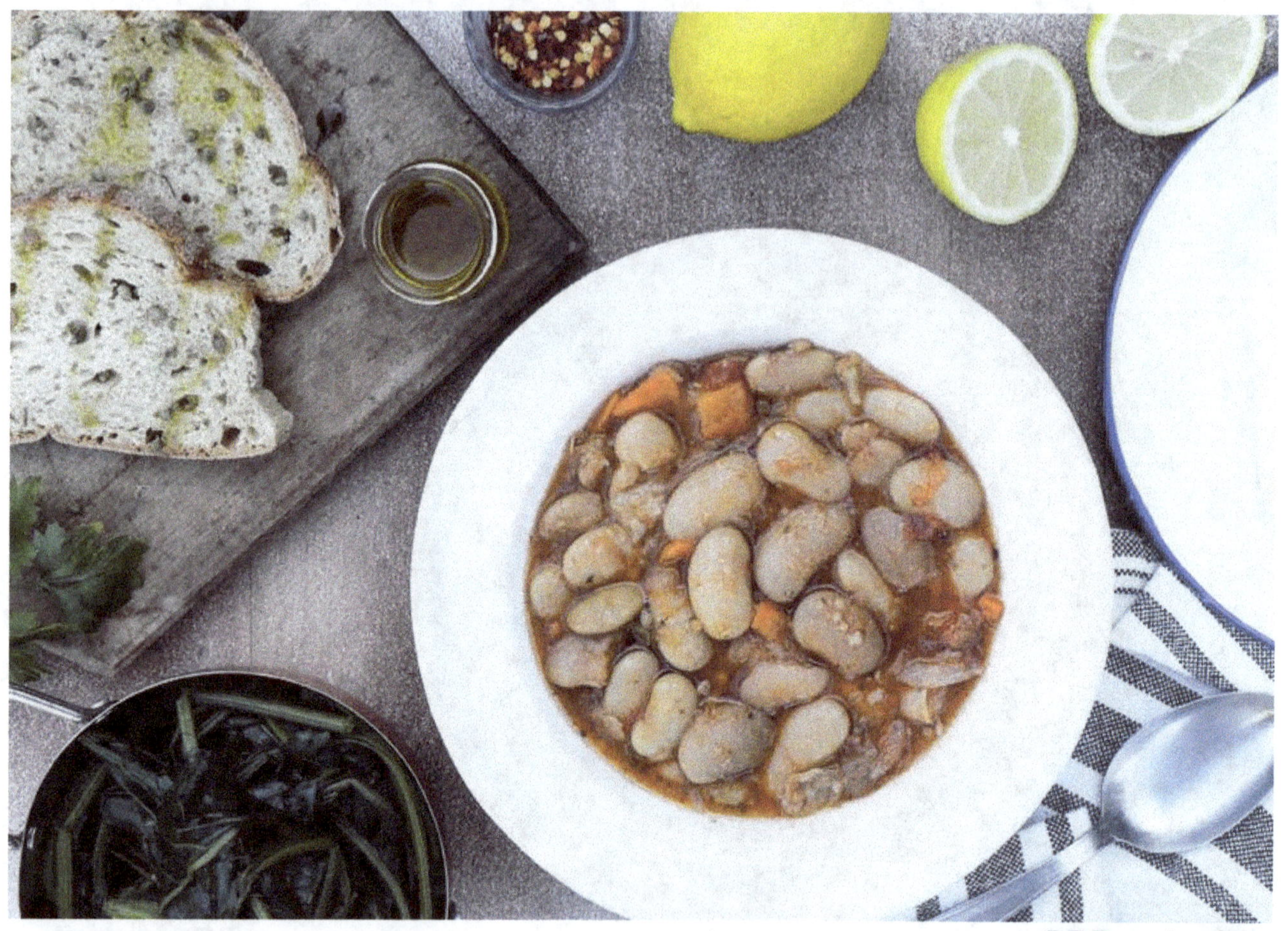

300 calories

What You'll Need:

- 1 cup fresh spinach
- 1 cup white beans
- 1 cup vegetable broth
- 1 onion, chopped
- 1 tbsp olive oil

Directions:

- Sauté onion in olive oil until translucent.
- Add white beans and vegetable broth.
- Simmer for 10 minutes.
- Stir in spinach until wilted

BROCCOLI CHEDDAR SOUP

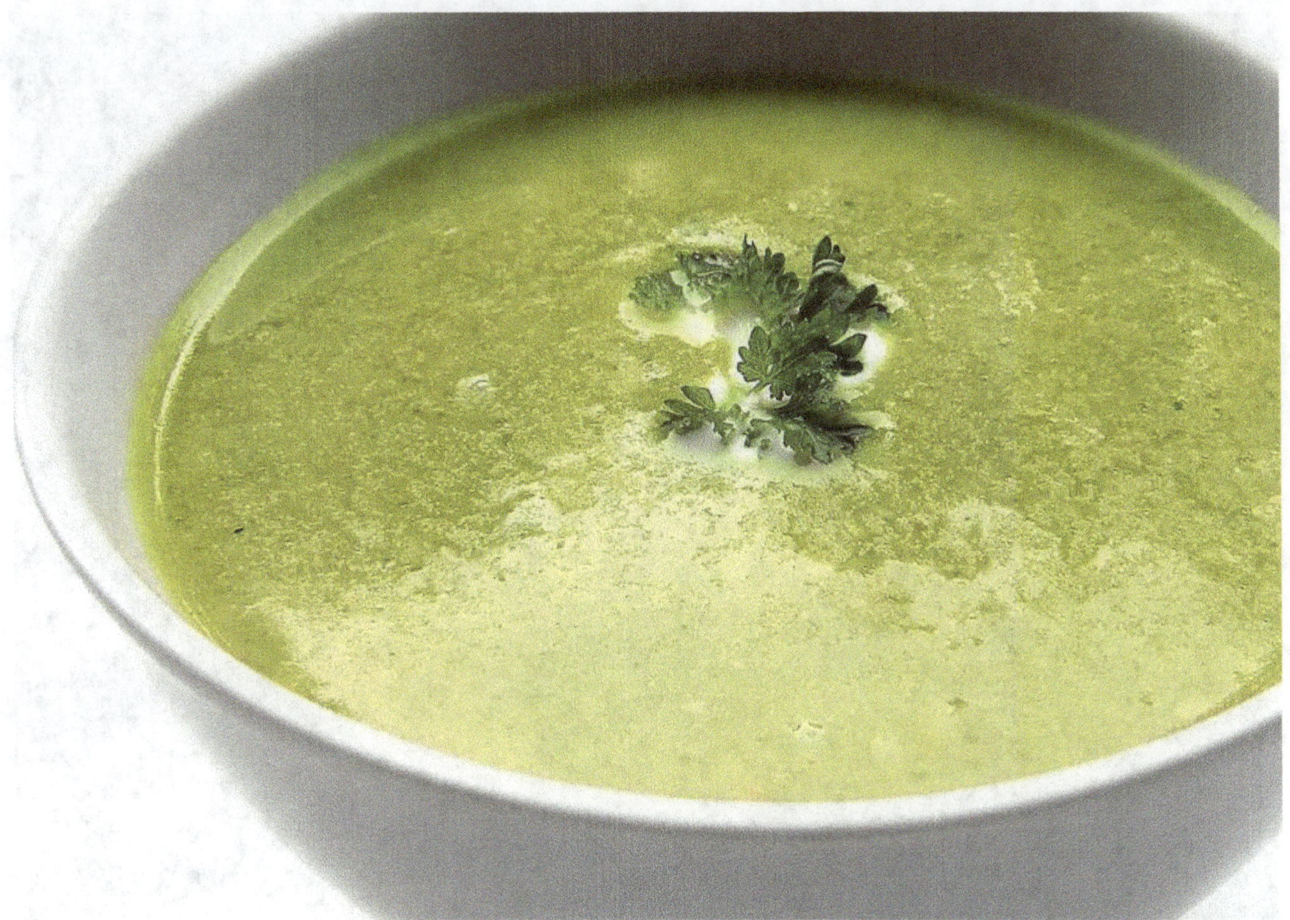

300 calories

What You'll Need:

- 2 cups broccoli florets
- 1 cup cheddar cheese, shredded
- 1 cup vegetable broth
- 1 cup milk
- 1 tbsp olive oil

Directions:

- Sauté broccoli in olive oil until tender.
- Add vegetable broth and milk and bring to a boil.
- Blend until smooth.
- Stir in cheddar cheese until melted and serve.

CHICKEN TORTILLA SOUP

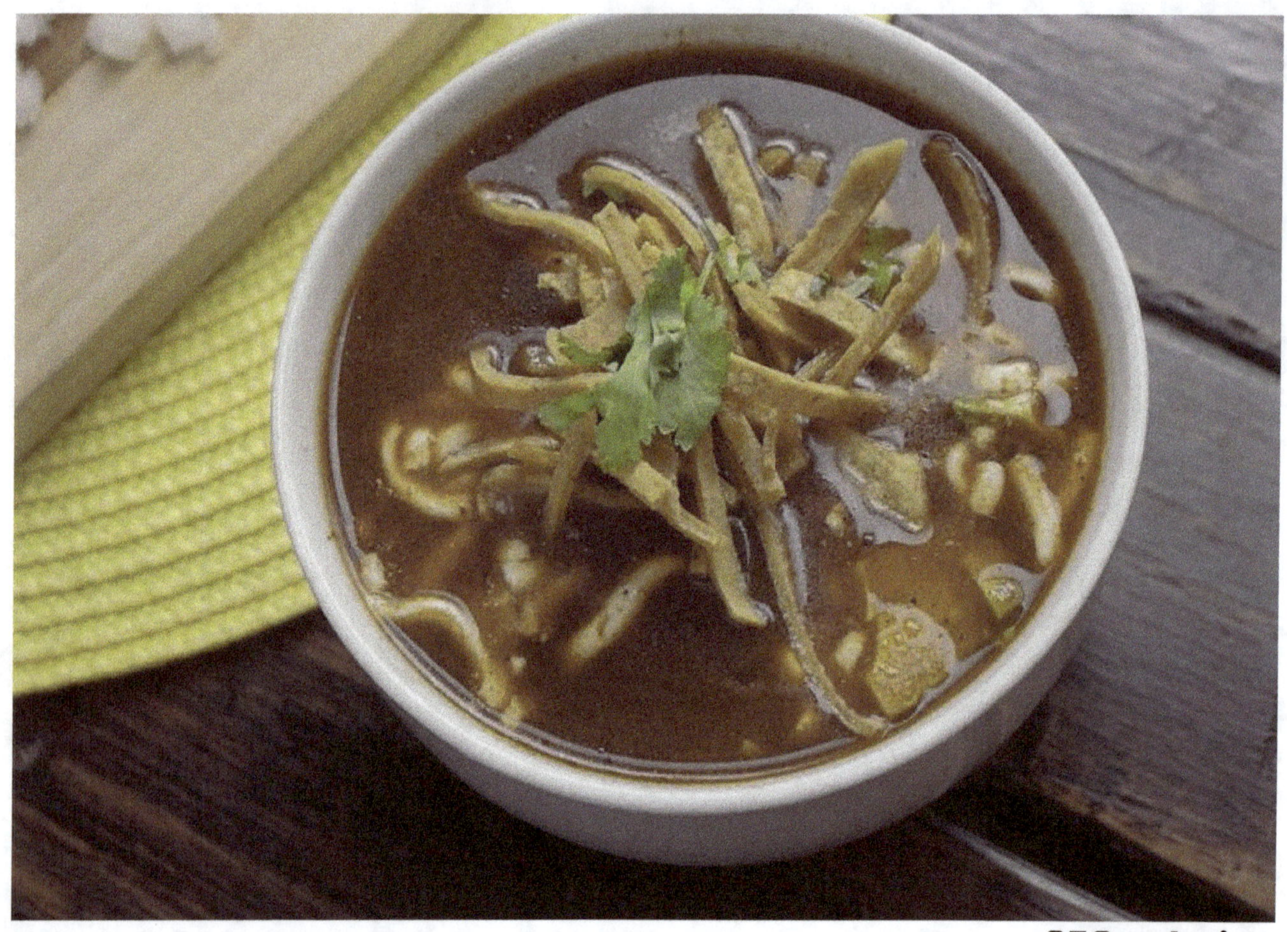

350 calories

<u>**What You'll Need:**</u>

- 1 cup cooked chicken breast, shredded
- 1 cup tortilla strips
- 1 cup diced tomatoes
- 1 cup chicken broth
- 1 tsp cumin

<u>**Directions:**</u>

- Combine chicken, tortilla strips, tomatoes, and chicken broth in a pot.
- Simmer until flavors are blended.
- Season with cumin and serve.

POTATO LEEK SOUP

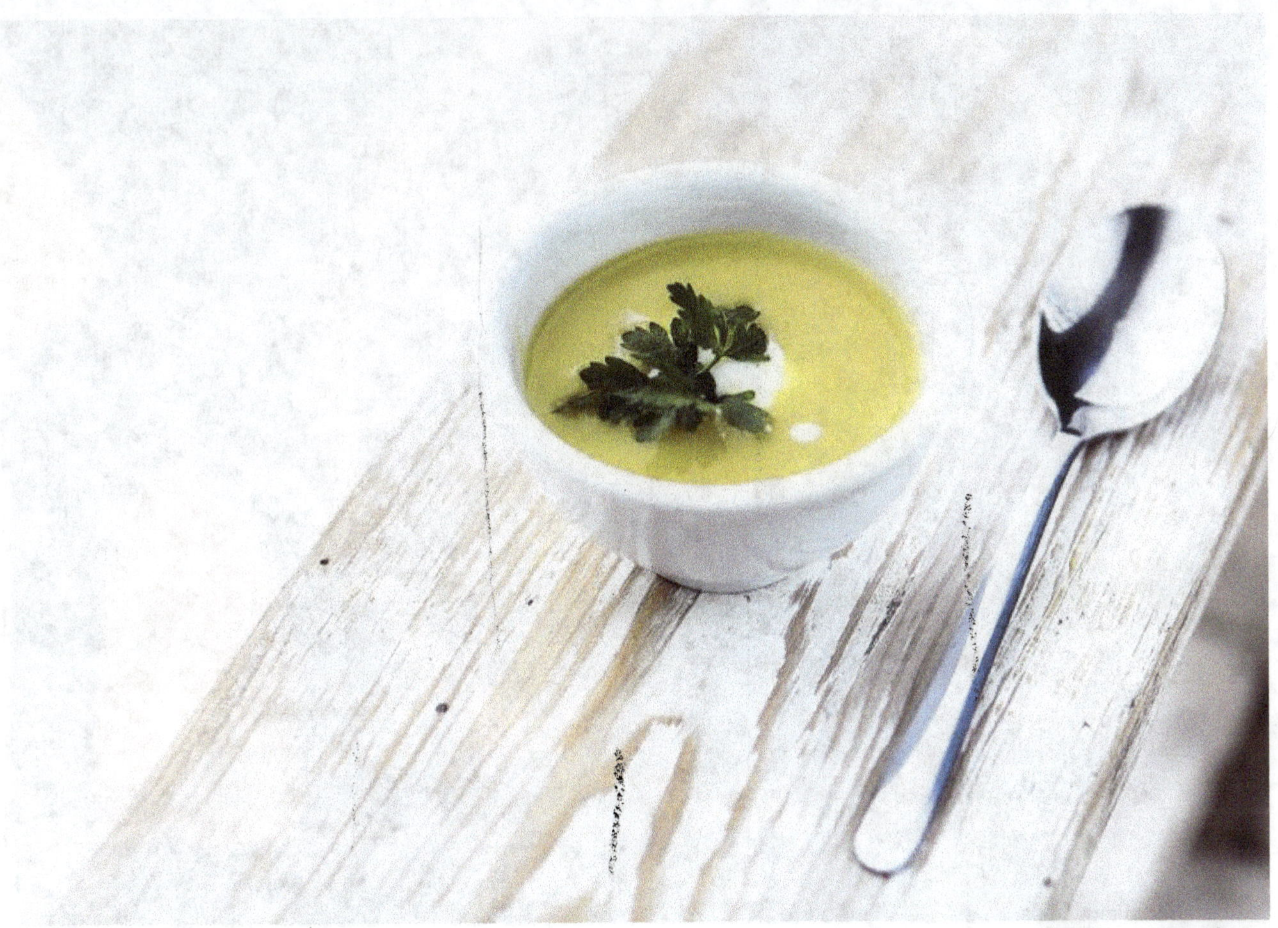

250 calories

What You'll Need:

- 2 cups potatoes, peeled and diced
- 1 cup leeks, chopped
- 1 cup vegetable broth
- 1 tbsp olive oil

Directions:

- Sauté leeks in olive oil until soft.
- Add potatoes and vegetable broth.
- Simmer until potatoes are tender.
- Blend until smooth and serve.

ROASTED RED PEPPER SOUP

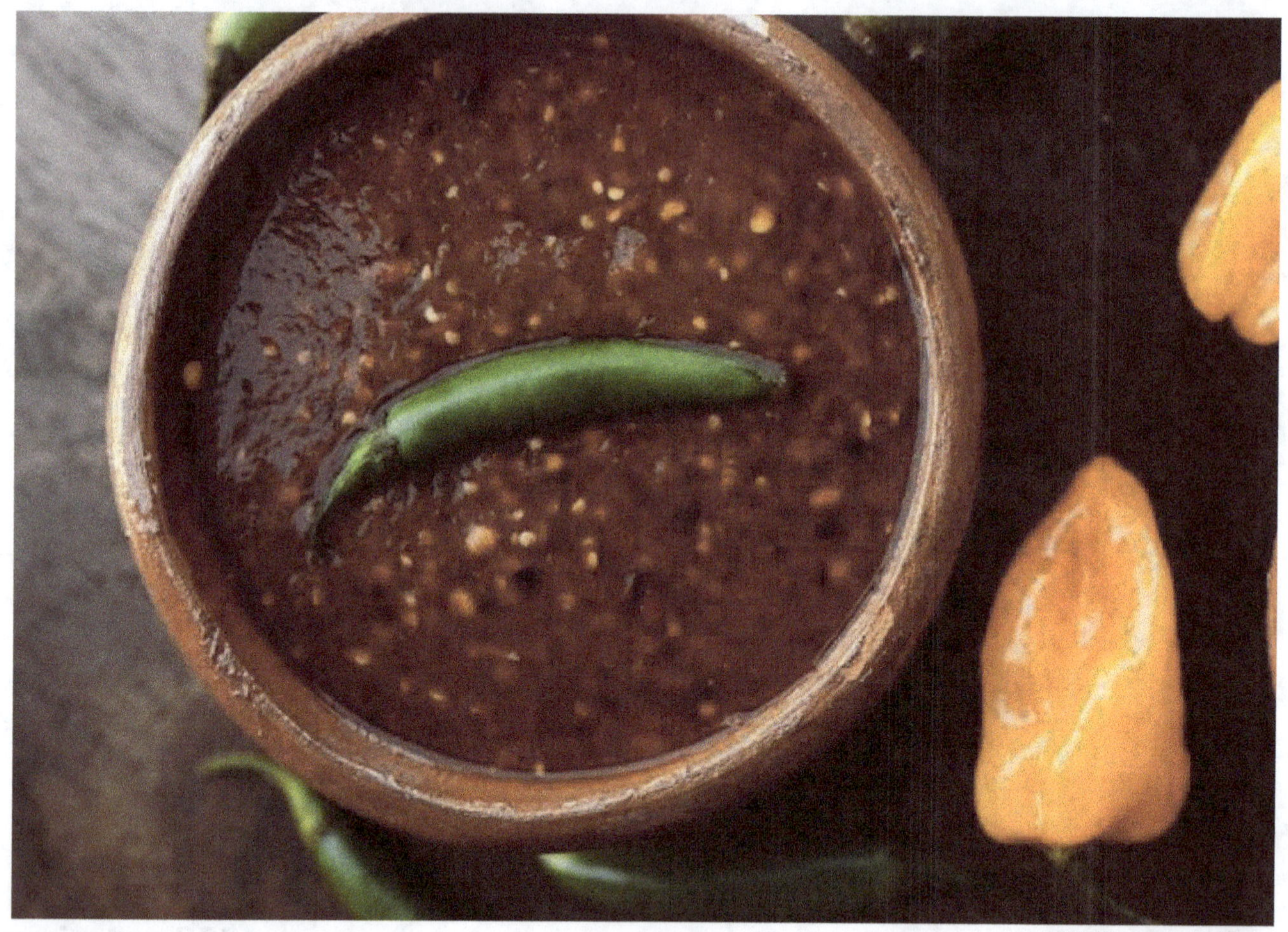

200 calories

<u>**What You'll Need:**</u>

- 2 cups roasted red peppers
- 1 cup vegetable broth
- 1 onion, chopped
- 1 tbsp olive oil

<u>**Directions:**</u>

- Sauté onion in olive oil until translucent.
- Add roasted red peppers and vegetable broth.
- Simmer for 15 minutes.
- Blend until smooth and serve.

CORN CHOWDER

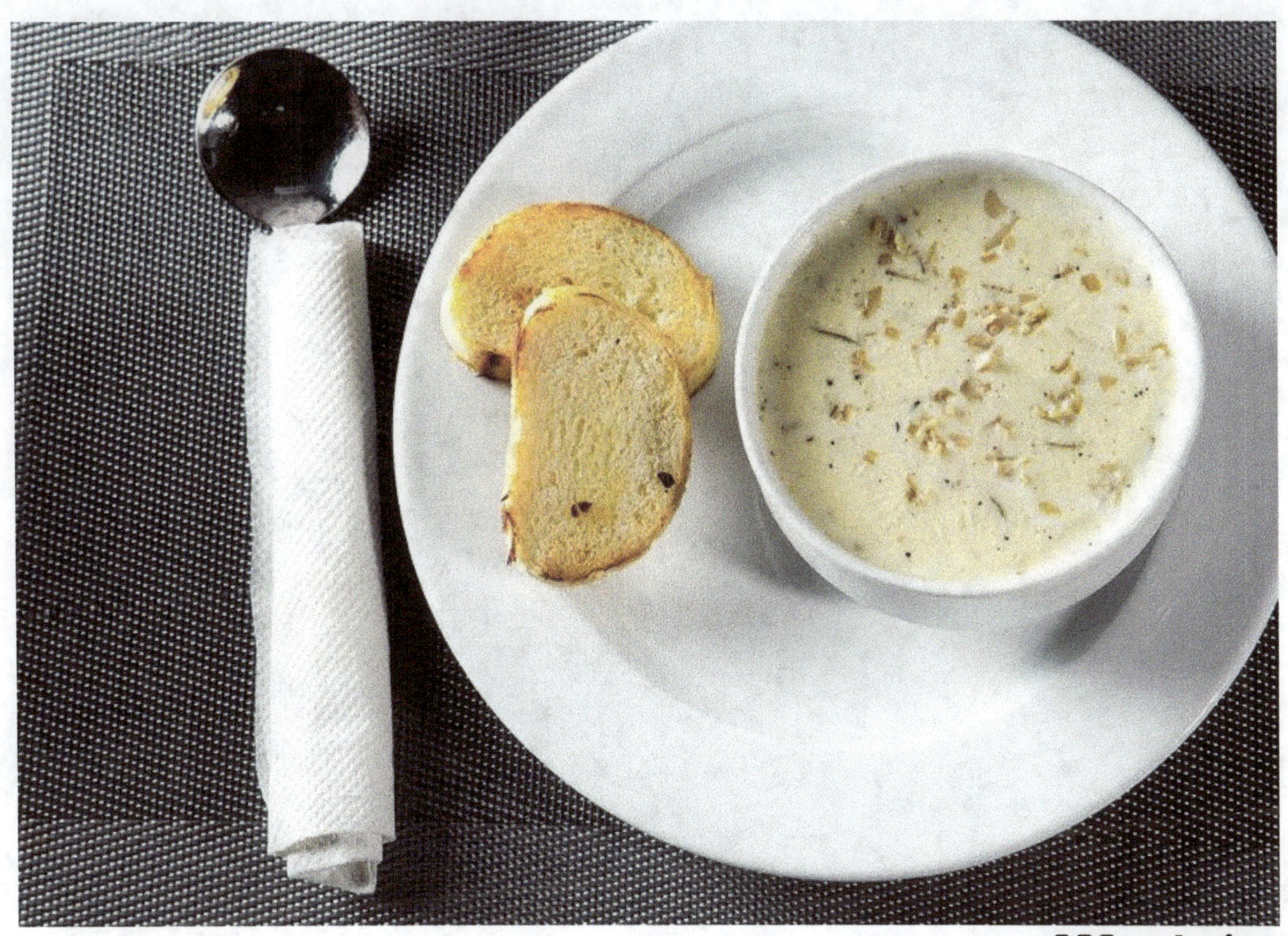

What You'll Need:

- 1 cup corn kernels
- 1 cup diced potatoes
- 1 cup vegetable broth
- 1 cup milk
- 1 tbsp butter

Directions:

- Sauté potatoes in butter until slightly tender.
- Add corn and vegetable broth.
- Simmer until potatoes are fully cooked.
- Stir in milk and season to taste.

GAZPACHO

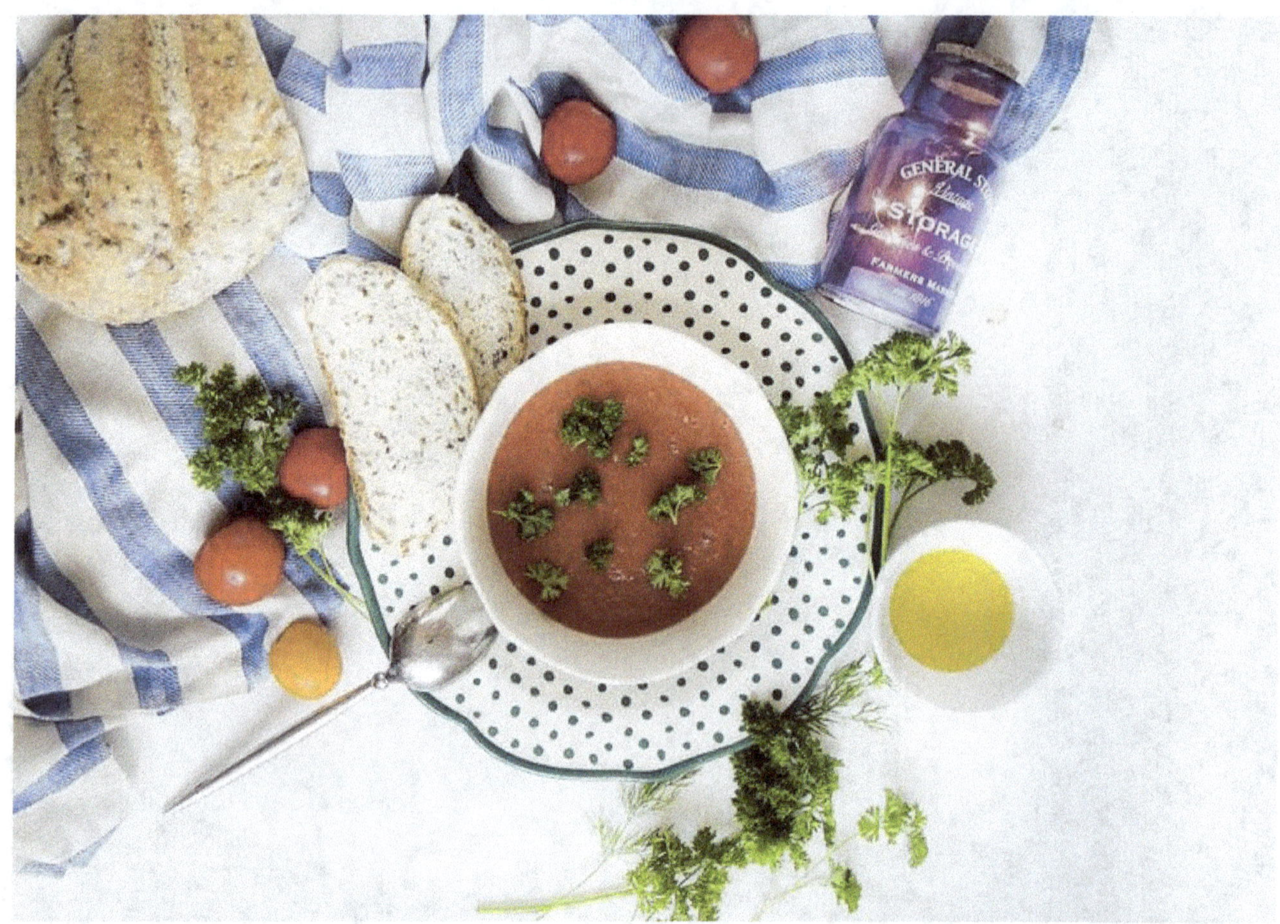

180 calories

What You'll Need:

- 2 cups tomatoes, chopped
- 1 cup cucumber, diced
- 1 cup bell peppers, diced
- 1 tbsp olive oil
- 1 tbsp vinegar

Directions:

- Combine tomatoes, cucumber, and bell peppers in a bowl.
- Stir in olive oil and vinegar.
- Chill for at least 2 hours before serving.

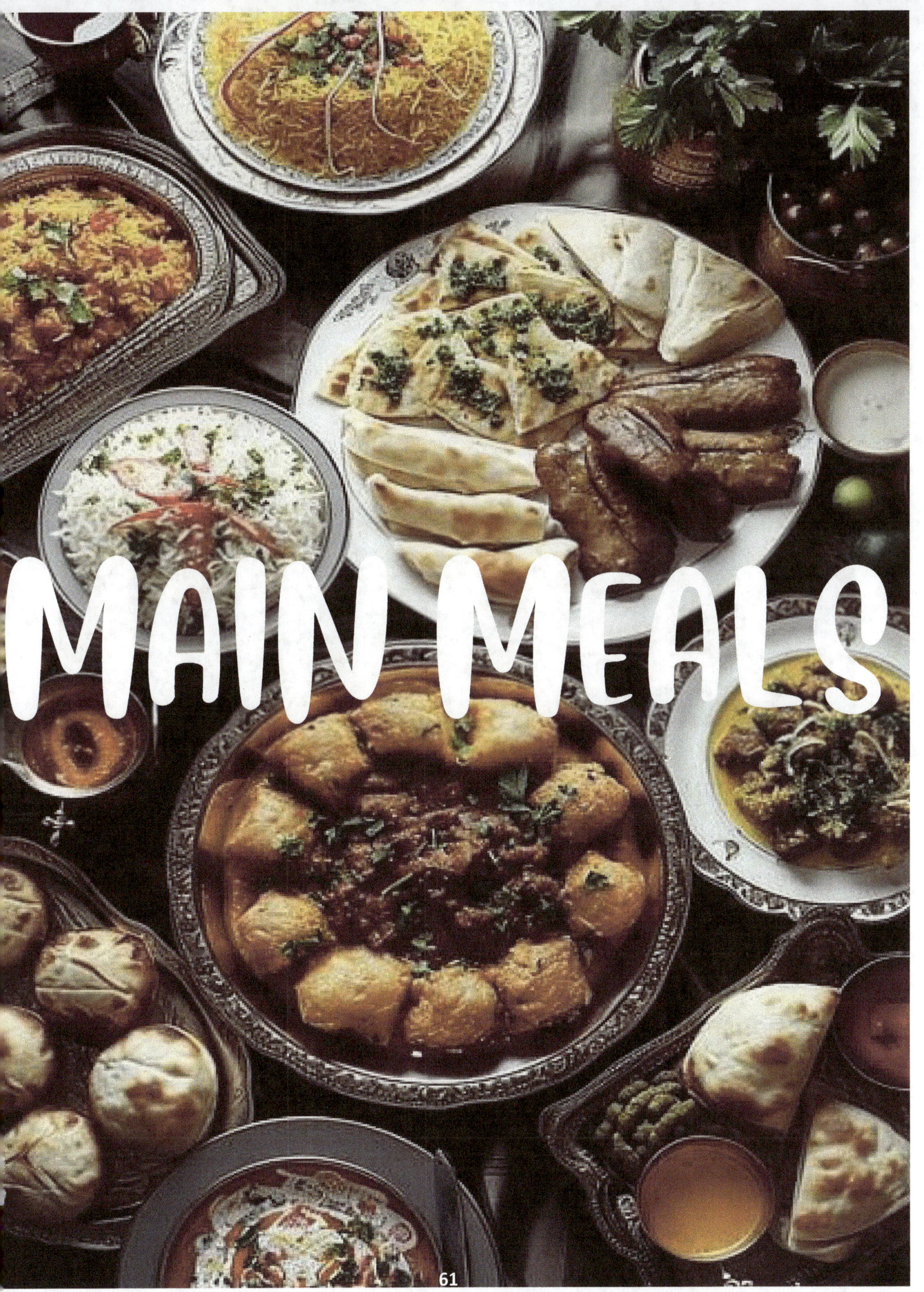

MAIN MEALS

BAKED SALMON WITH LEMON

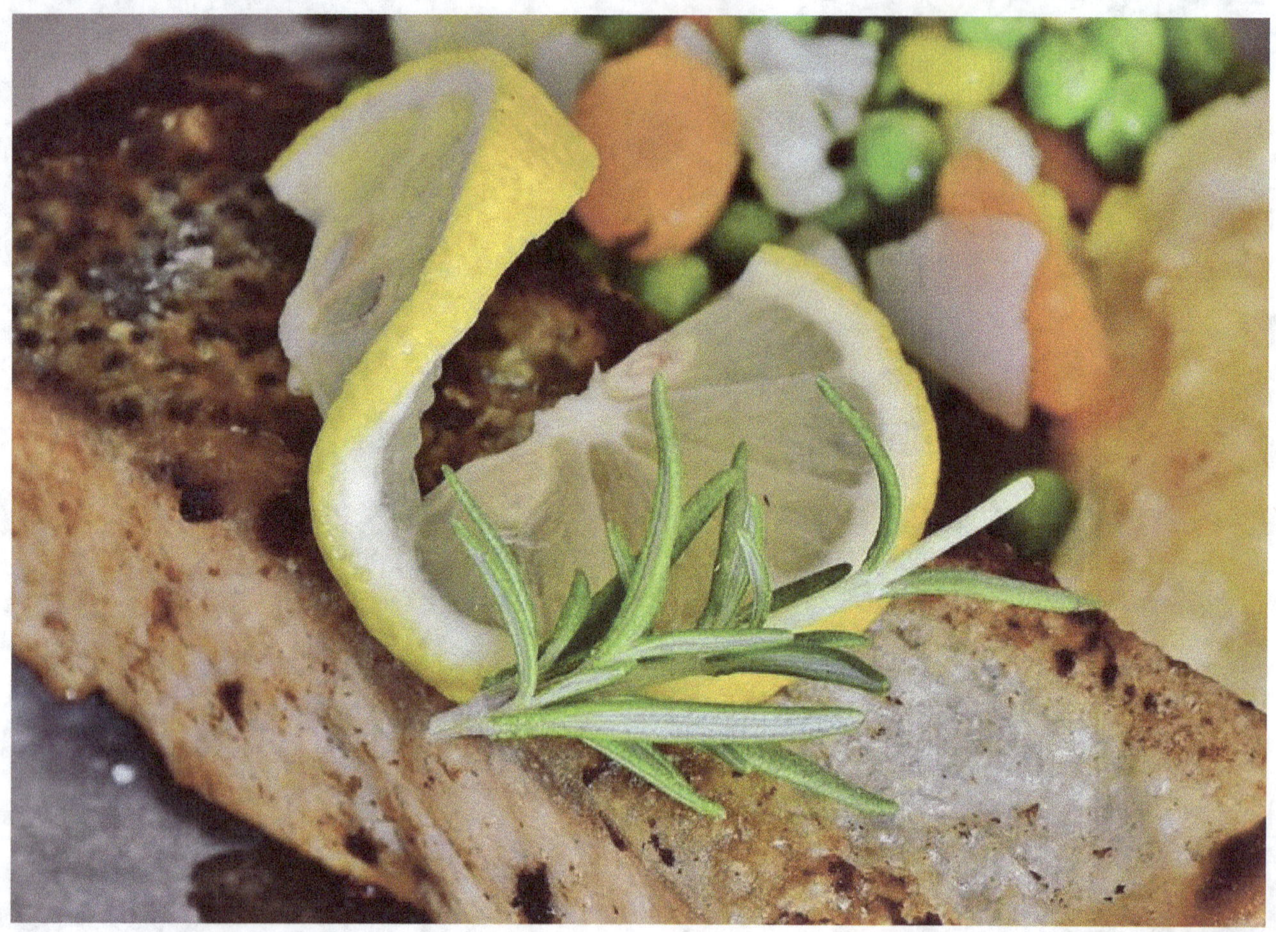

400 calories

What You'll Need:

- 4 oz salmon fillet
- 1 lemon, sliced
- 1 tsp dill
- 1 tbsp olive oil

Directions:

- Preheat oven to 400°F (200°C).
- Place salmon on a baking sheet.
- Drizzle with olive oil and season with dill.
- Top with lemon slices.
- Bake for 15–20 minutes.

STUFFED BELL PEPPERS

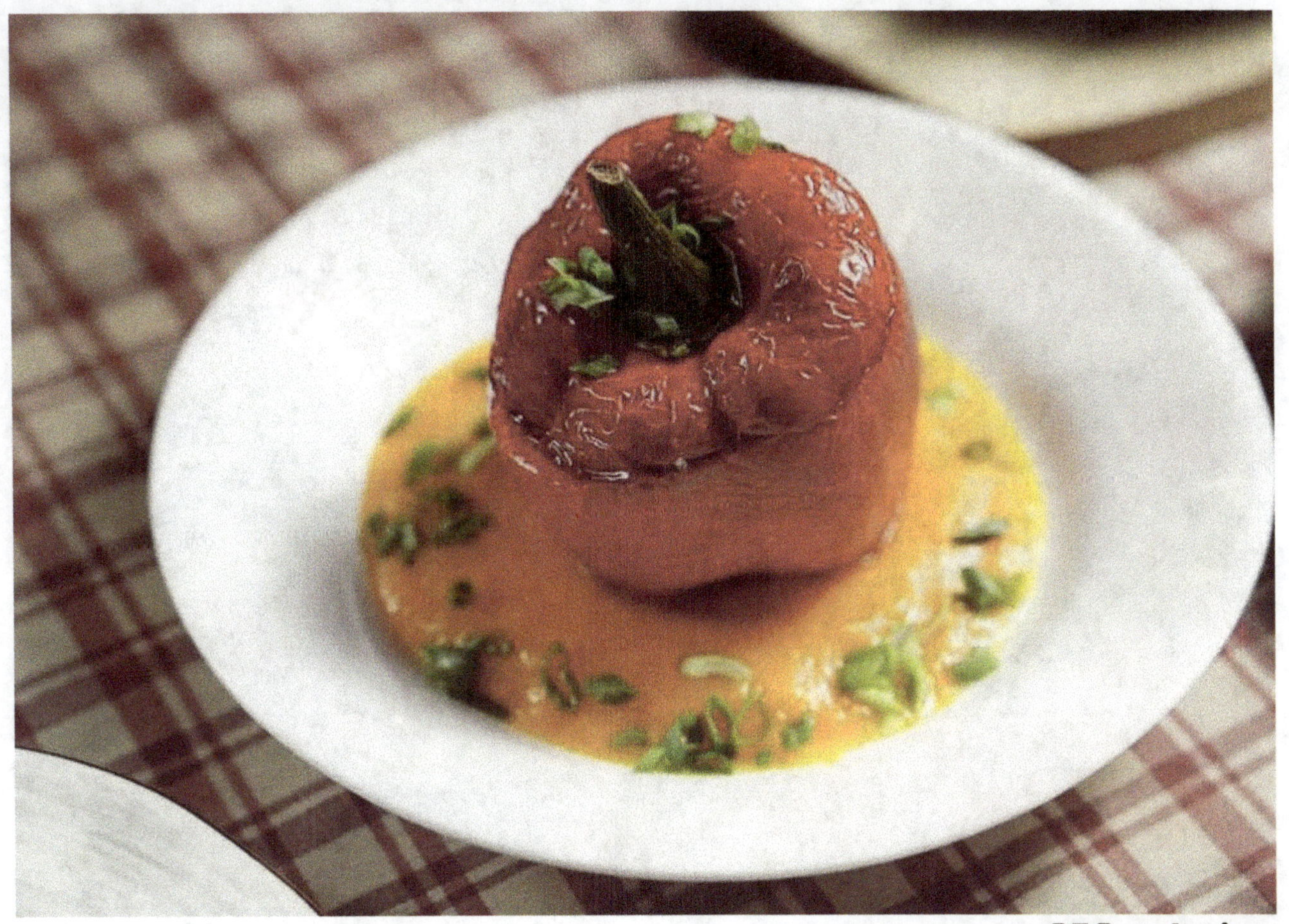

350 calories

What You'll Need:

- 2 bell peppers
- 1 cup cooked quinoa
- ½ cup black beans
- ¼ cup corn
- 1 tsp cumin

Directions:

- Preheat oven to 375°F (190°C).
- Mix quinoa, black beans, corn, and cumin.
- Stuff bell peppers with the mixture.
- Bake for 30–35 minutes.

CHICKEN STIR-FRY

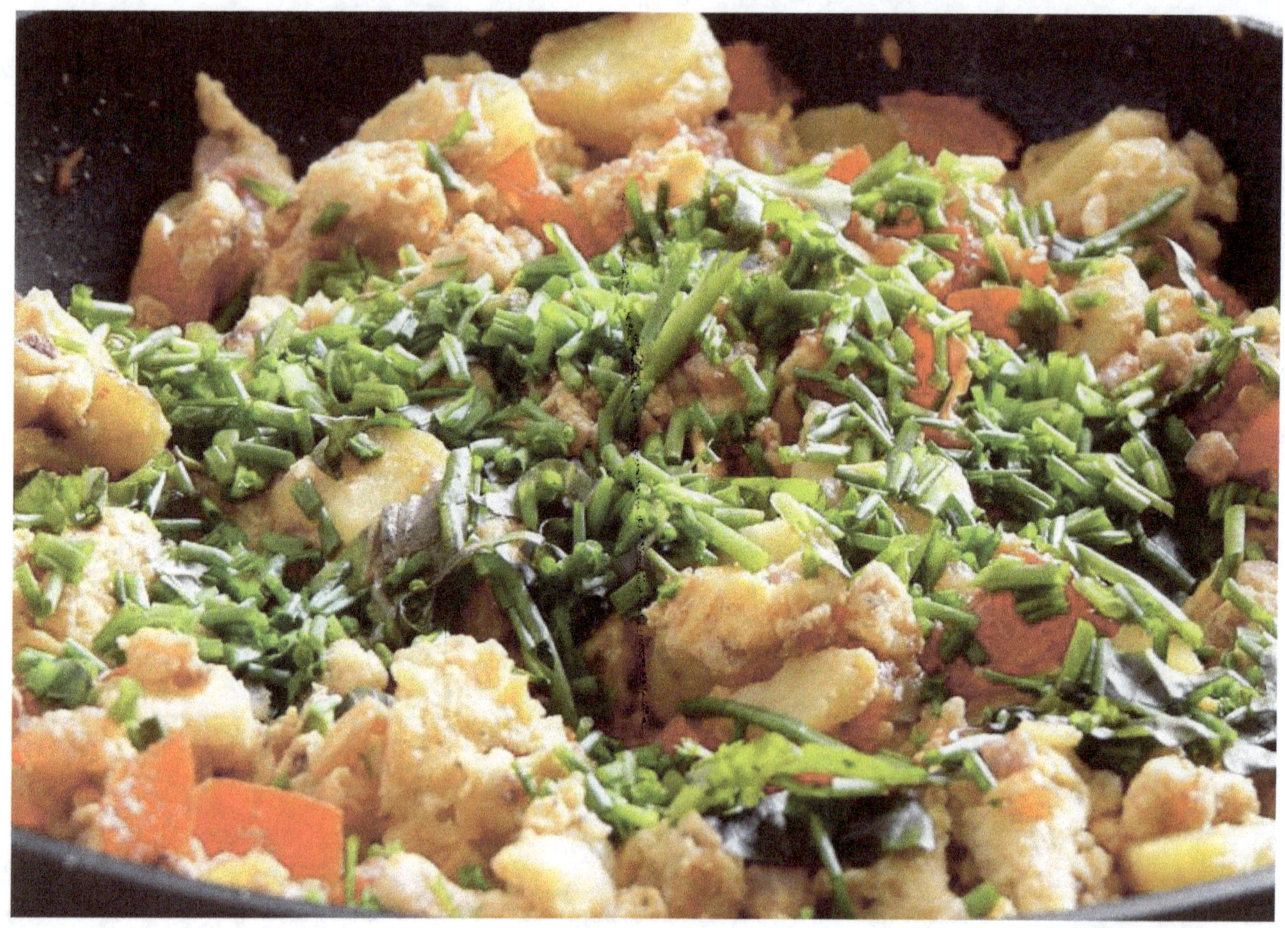

What You'll Need:

- 3 oz chicken breast, sliced
- 1 cup mixed vegetables (broccoli, bell peppers, snap peas)
- 2 tbsp soy sauce
- 1 tbsp olive oil

Directions:

- Sauté chicken in olive oil until cooked through.
- Add vegetables and stir-fry until tender.
- Stir in soy sauce and serve.

SWEET POTATO AND BLACK BEAN CHILI

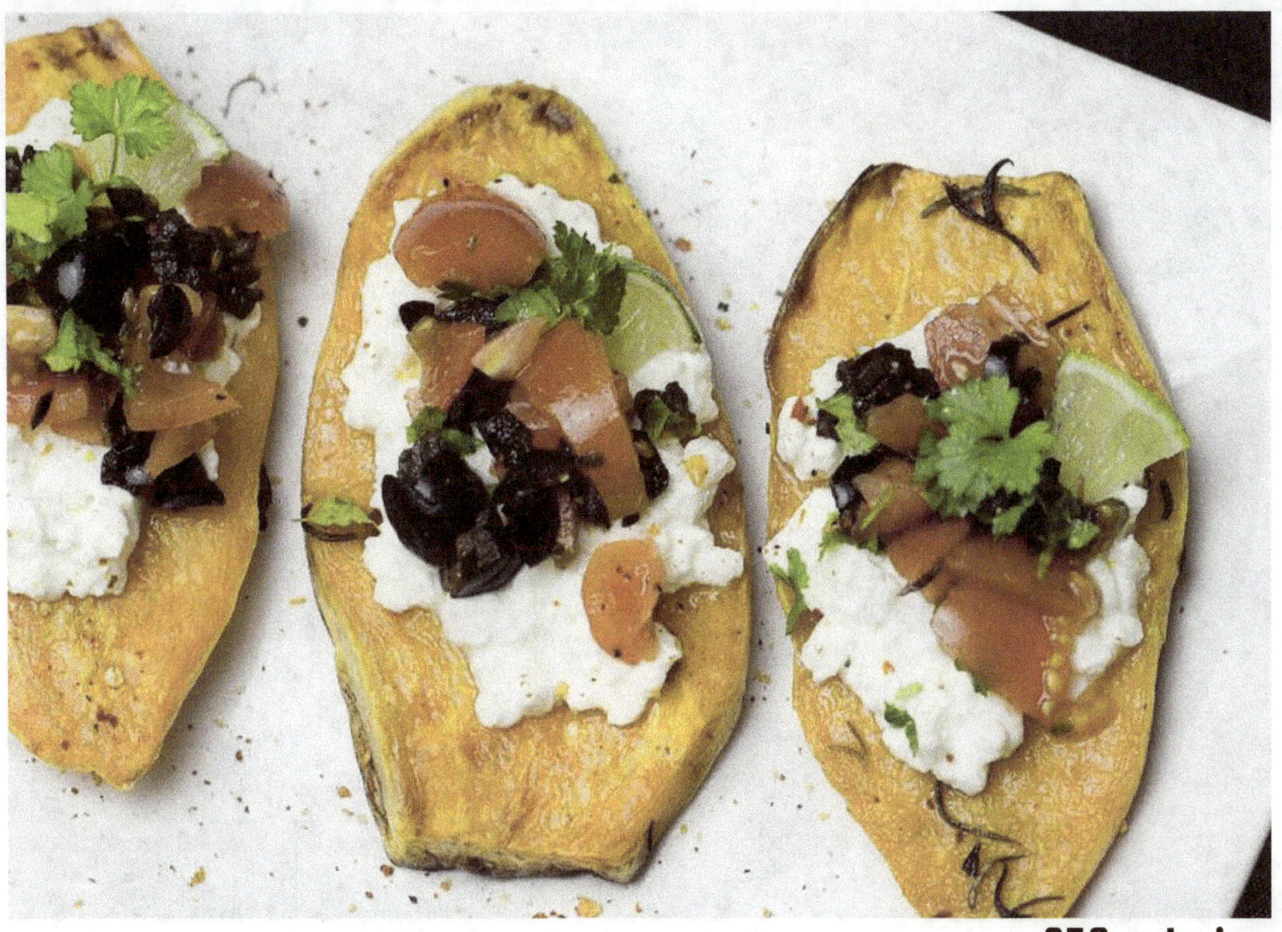

350 calories

What You'll Need:

- 1 cup sweet potatoes, diced
- 1 cup black beans
- 1 cup diced tomatoes
- 1 cup vegetable broth
- 1 tsp chili powder

Directions:

- Sauté sweet potatoes in a pot until slightly tender.
- Add black beans, diced tomatoes, vegetable broth, and chili powder.
- Simmer until sweet potatoes are fully cooked.
- Season to taste and serve.

GRILLED CHICKEN WITH RICE

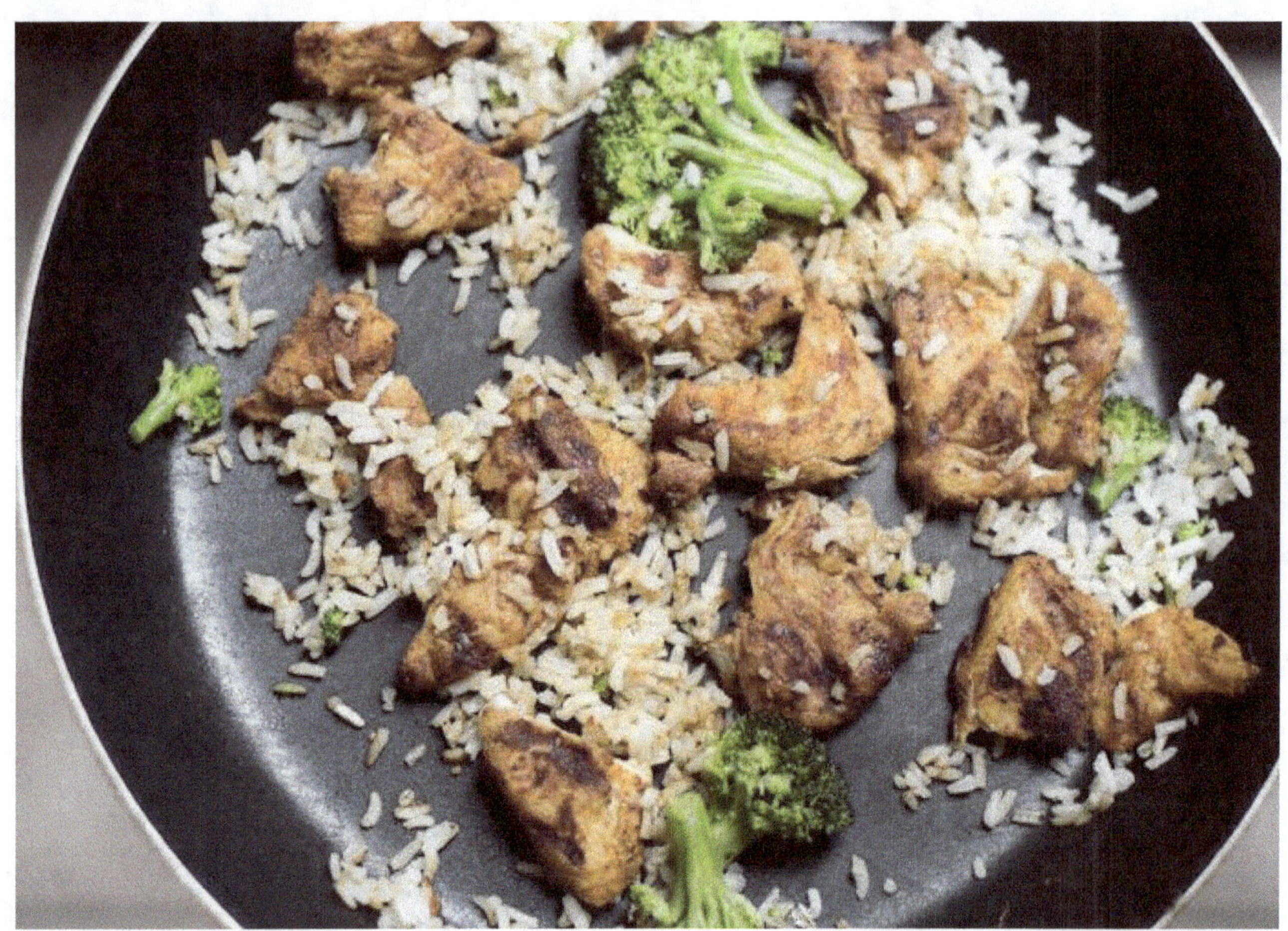

What You'll Need:

- 4 oz chicken breast
- 1 cup cooked rice
- 1 tbsp olive oil
- 1 tsp paprika

Directions:

- Cook the rice according to the package instructions.
- Heat the olive oil in a skillet over medium heat.
- Add the chicken breast to the skillet and sprinkle with paprika.
- Cook the chicken until it's fully cooked, then serve it with the rice.

SPAGHETTI SQUASH WITH MARINARA

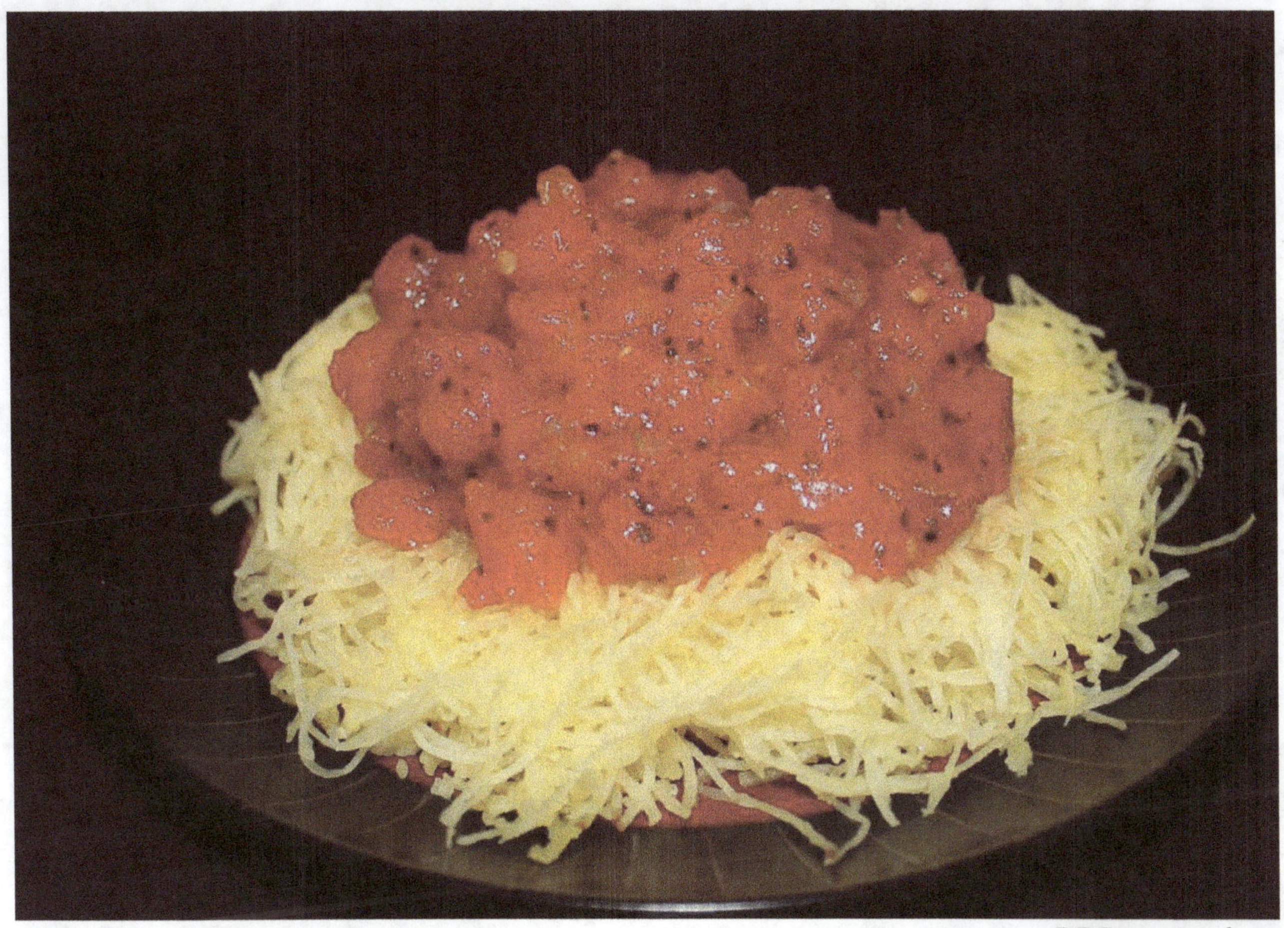

300 calories

What You'll Need:

- 1 medium spaghetti squash
- 1 cup marinara sauce
- 1 tbsp olive oil
- 1 tsp Italian seasoning

Directions:

- Preheat oven to 400°F (200°C).
- Cut squash in half and remove seeds.
- Drizzle with olive oil and roast for 40-45 minutes.
- Scrape squash strands with a fork and top with marinara sauce.
- Sprinkle with Italian seasoning and serve

SHRIMP TACOS

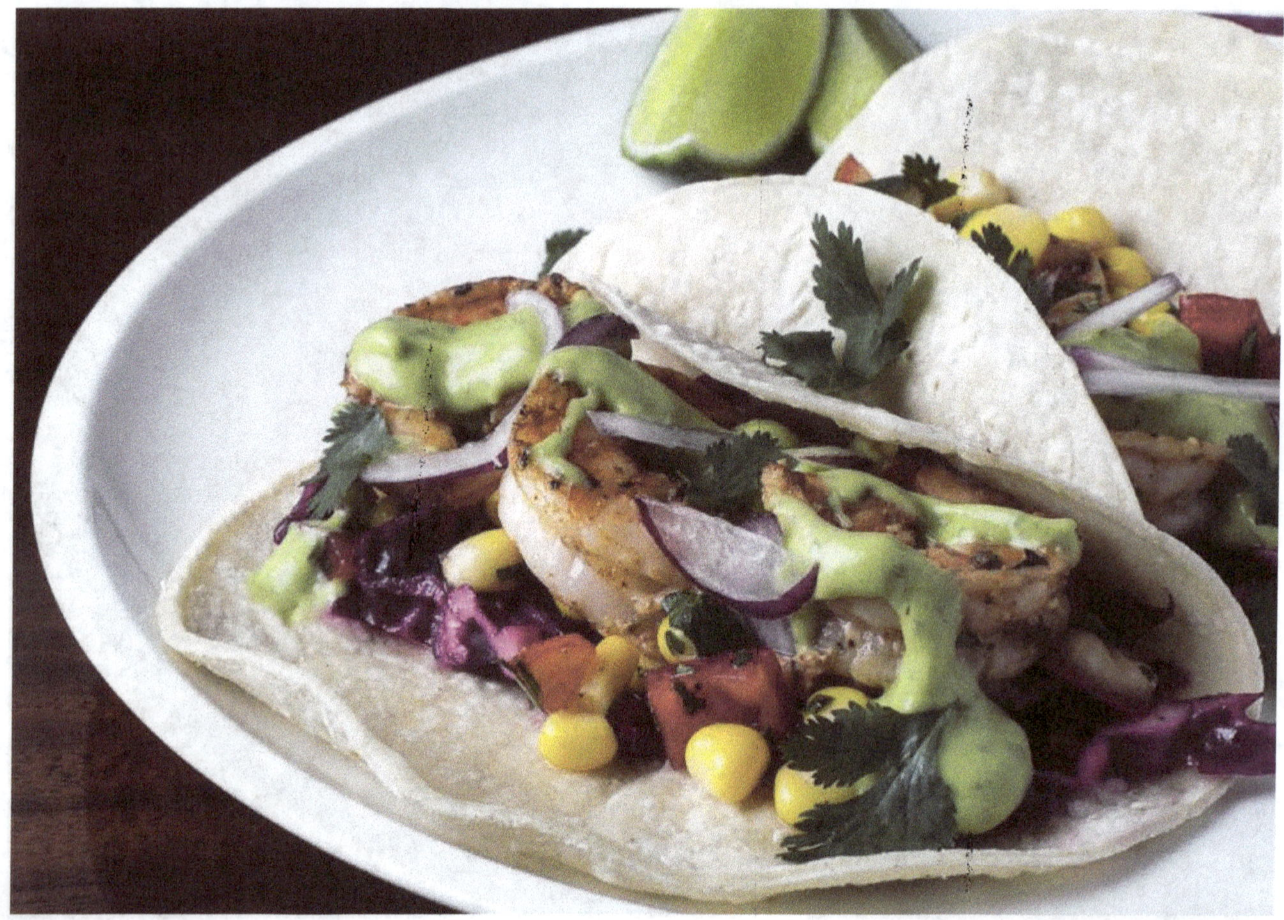

350 calories

What You'll Need:

- 4 oz shrimp, peeled and deveined
- 2 small tortillas
- ½ cup shredded cabbage
- 2 tbsp salsa
- 1 tbsp lime juice

Directions:

- Sauté shrimp in a pan until cooked through.
- Warm tortillas and fill with shrimp, shredded cabbage, salsa, and lime juice.
- Serve immediately.

VEGETABLE CURRY

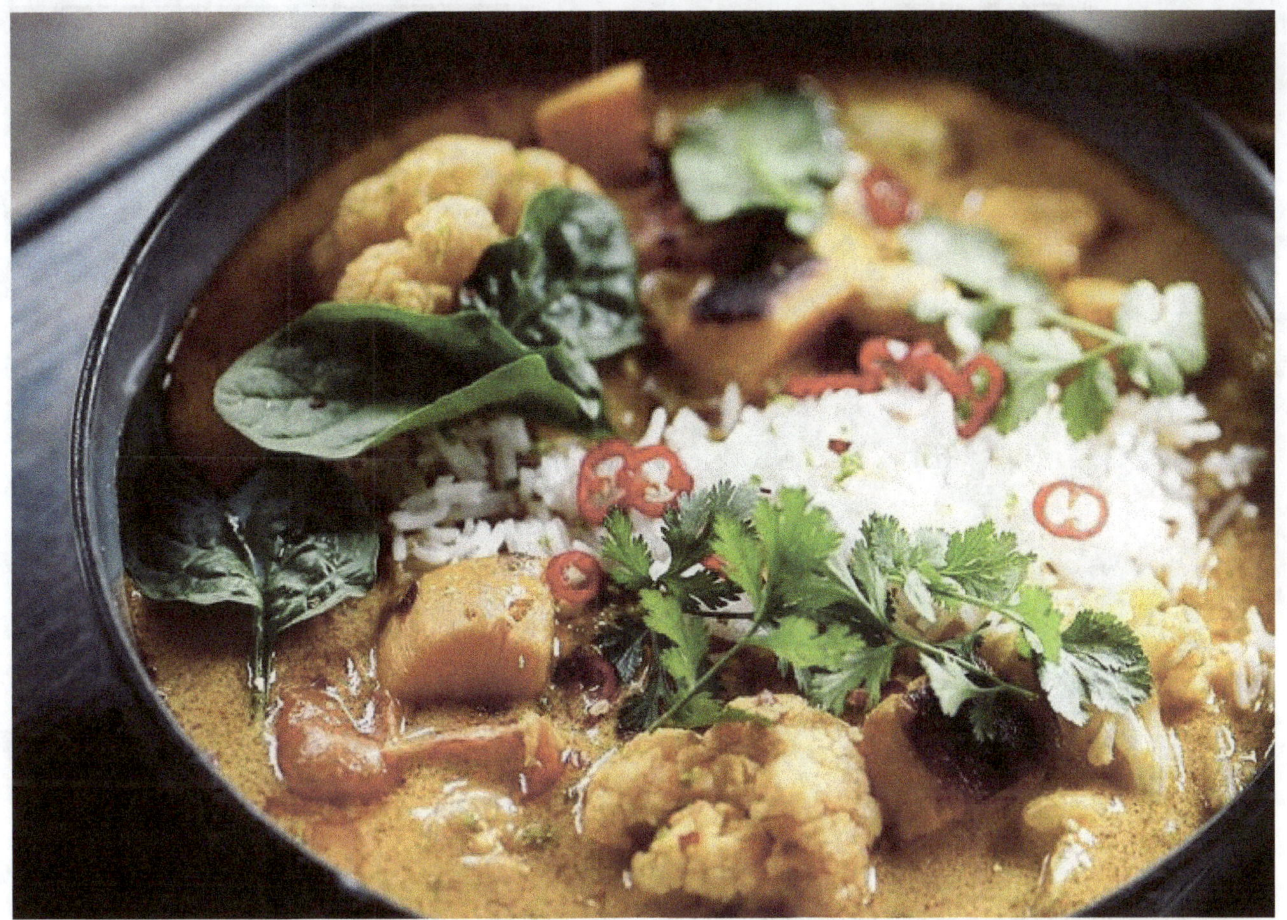

300 calories

What You'll Need:

- 1 cup mixed vegetables (carrots, potatoes, bell peppers)
- 1 cup coconut milk
- 2 tbsp curry powder
- 1 tbsp olive oil

Directions:

- Sauté vegetables in olive oil until tender.
- Add coconut milk and curry powder.
- Simmer until vegetables are fully cooked.
- Serve with rice or naan.

TURKEY MEATBALLS

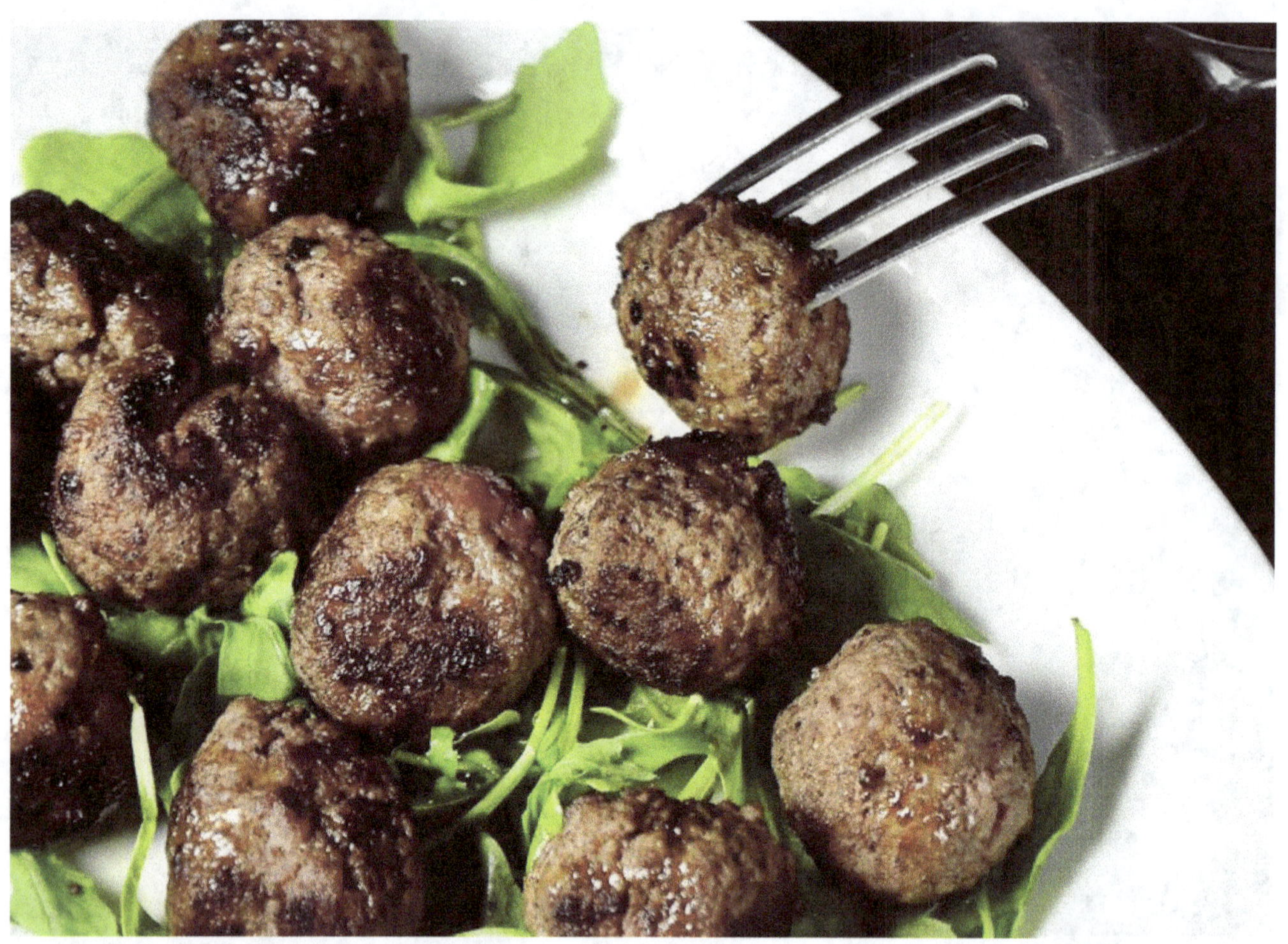

400 calories

What You'll Need:

- 4 oz ground turkey
- 1 egg
- ¼ cup breadcrumbs
- 1 tsp Italian seasoning
- 1 cup marinara sauce

Directions:

- Preheat oven to 375°F (190°C).
- Mix ground turkey with egg, breadcrumbs, and Italian seasoning.
- Form into meatballs and bake for 20–25 minutes.
- Simmer in marinara sauce before serving.

VEGETABLE LASAGNA

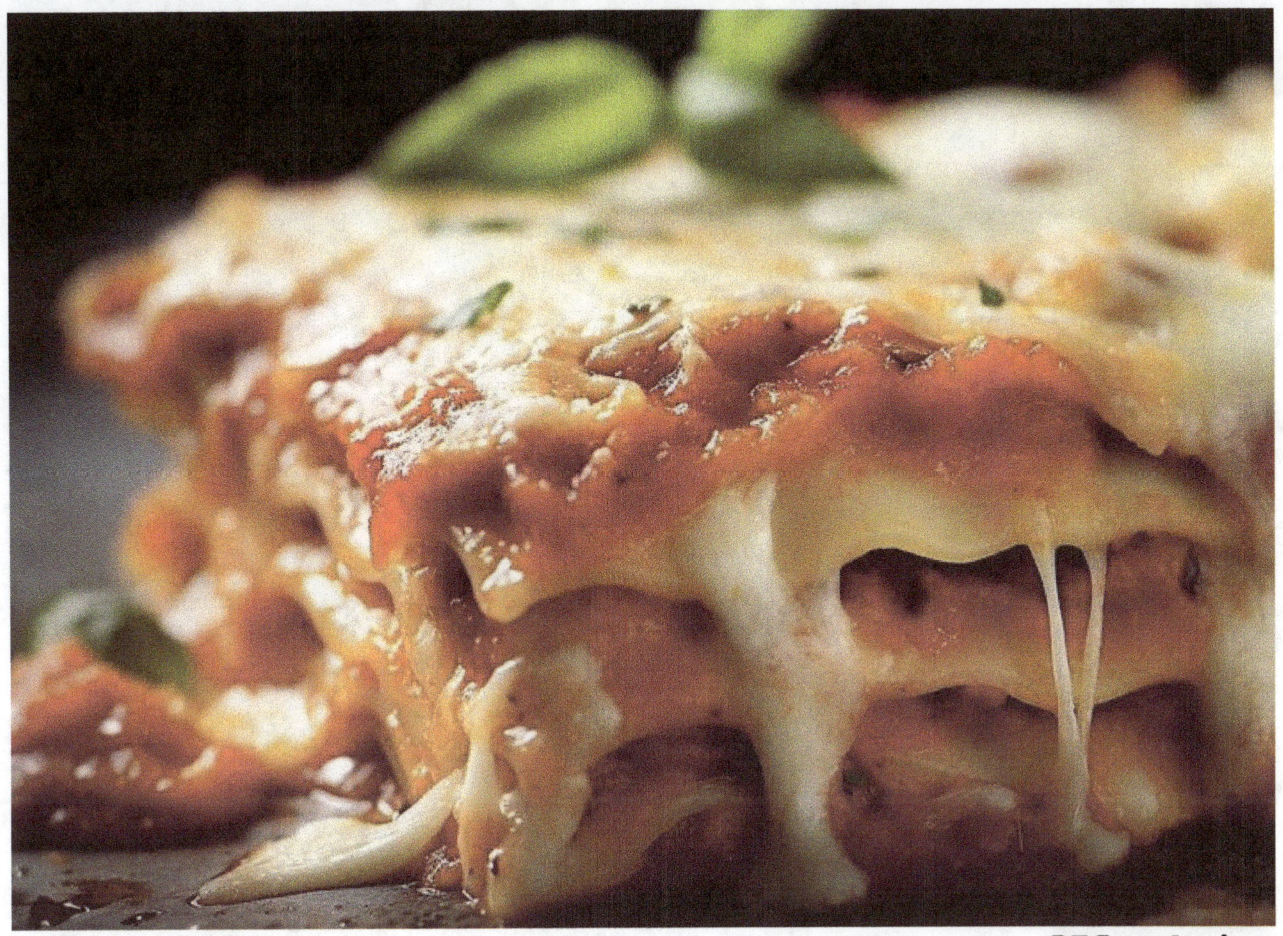

350 calories

What You'll Need:

- 2 cups ricotta cheese
- 1 cup spinach
- 1 cup marinara sauce
- 9 lasagna noodles
- 1 cup shredded mozzarella cheese

Directions:

- Preheat oven to 375°F (190°C).
- Cook lasagna noodles according to package instructions.
- Layer noodles, ricotta cheese, spinach, marinara sauce, and mozzarella cheese in a baking dish.
- Bake for 30–35 minutes.

GRILLED VEGGIE SKEWERS

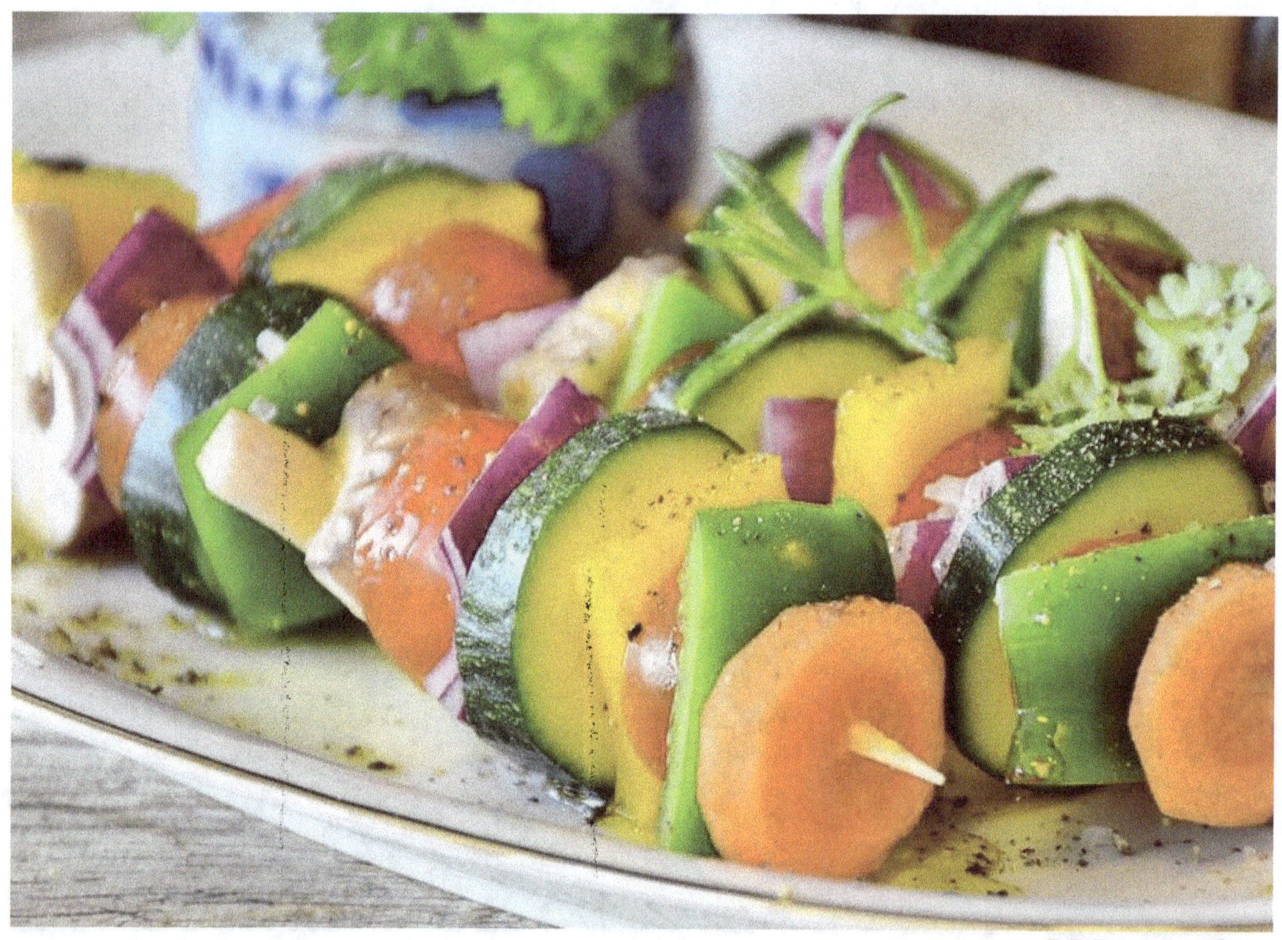

200 calories

What You'll Need:

- 1 cup mixed vegetables (bell peppers, zucchini, mushrooms)
- 1 tbsp olive oil
- 1 tsp garlic powder

Directions:

- Preheat grill to medium-high heat.
- Thread vegetables onto skewers.
- Brush with olive oil and sprinkle with garlic powder.
- Grill for 10-15 minutes, turning occasionally.

LEMON HERB CHICKEN

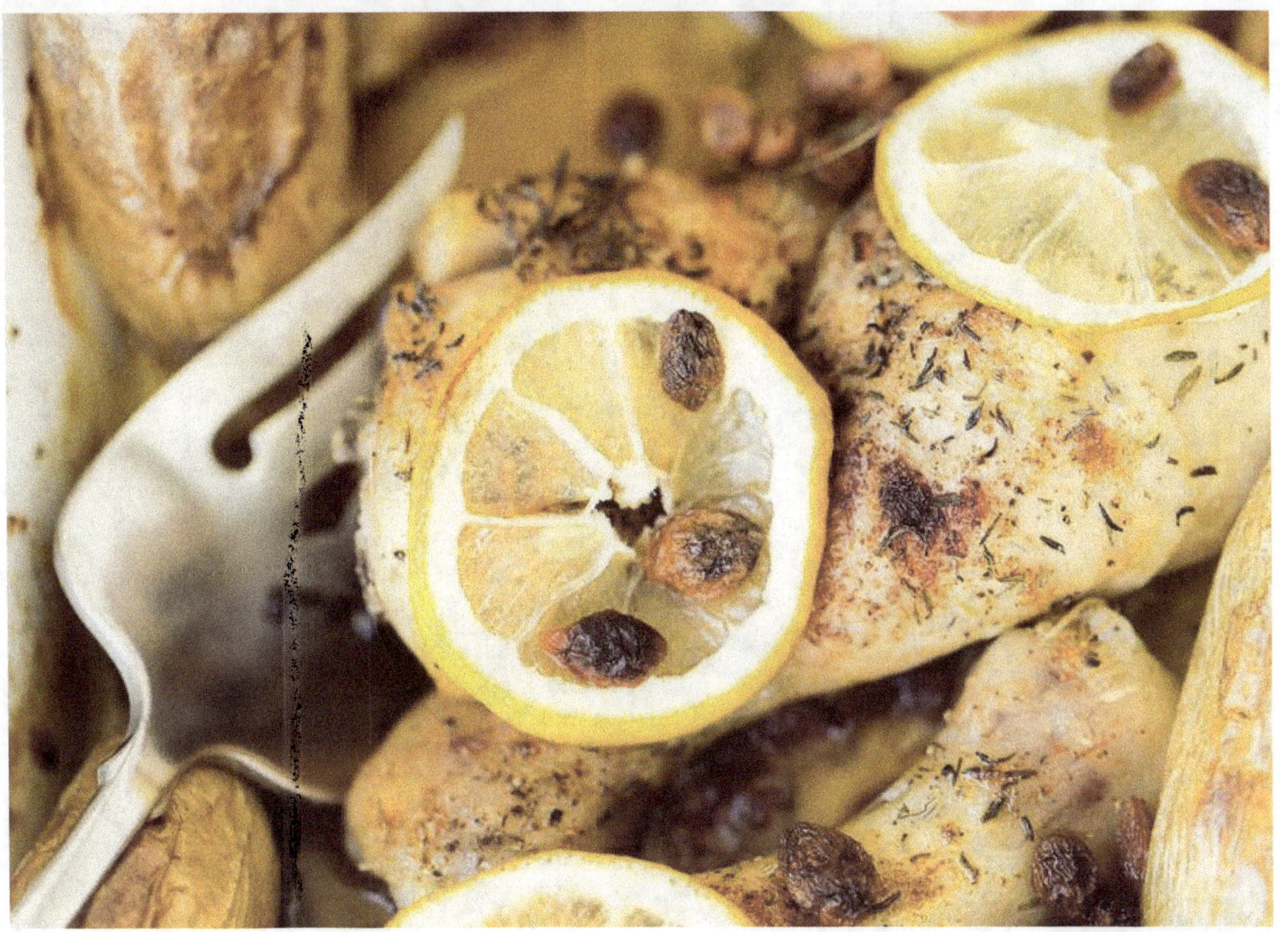

350 calories

What You'll Need:

- 4 oz chicken breast
- 1 lemon, juiced
- 1 tbsp olive oil
- 1 tsp mixed herbs (e.g., thyme, rosemary)

Directions:

- Preheat oven to 375°F (190°C).
- Marinate chicken in lemon juice, olive oil, and mixed herbs.
- Bake for 20–25 minutes, or until cooked through.

STUFFED ZUCCHINI BOATS

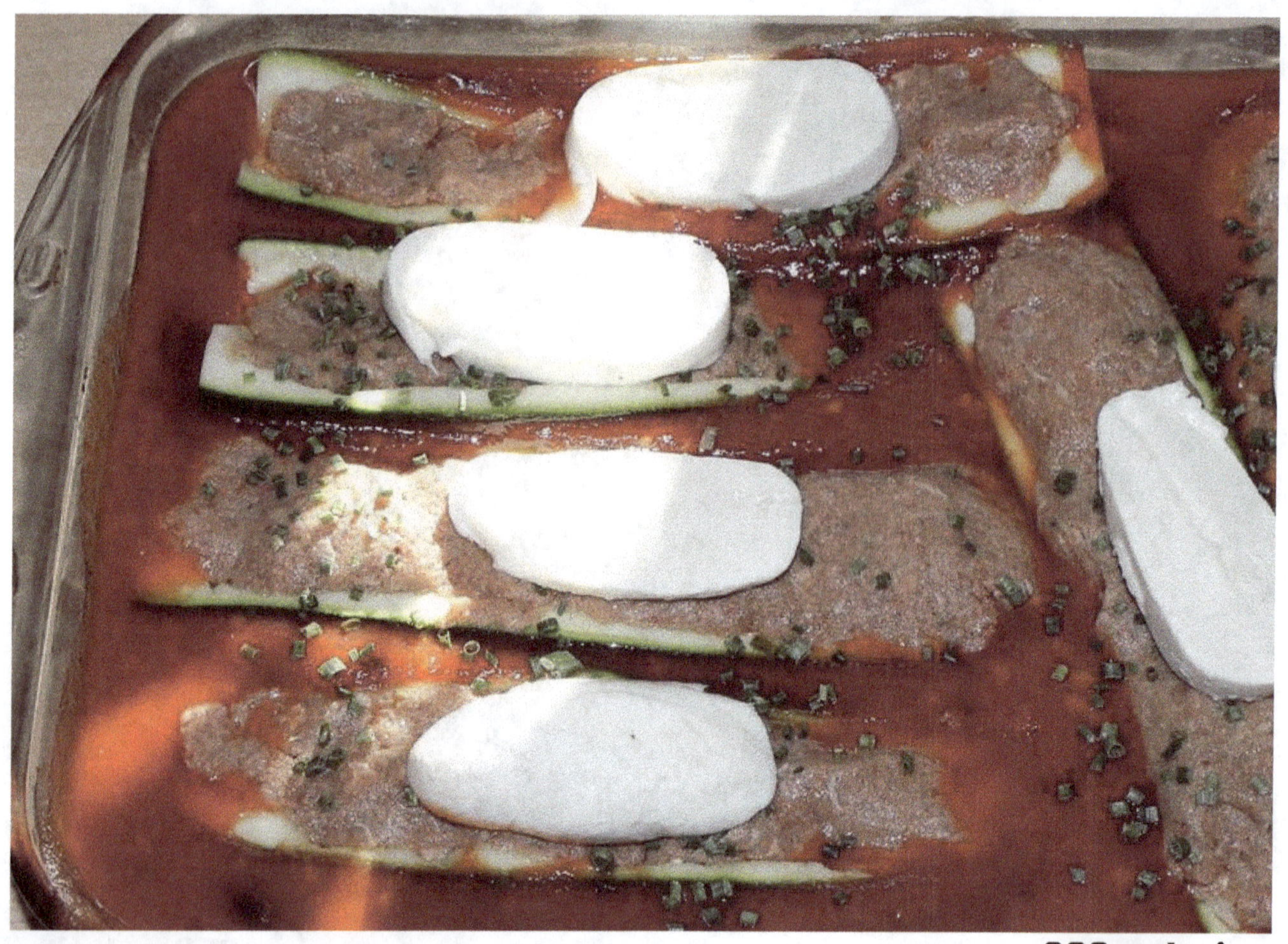

300 calories

What You'll Need:

- 2 medium zucchinis
- 1 cup cooked ground turkey
- ½ cup marinara sauce
- ¼ cup shredded mozzarella cheese

Directions:

- Preheat oven to 375°F (190°C).
- Slice zucchinis in half lengthwise and scoop out the seeds.
- Fill with ground turkey and marinara sauce.
- Top with mozzarella cheese and bake for 25–30 minutes.

AIR FRYER CHICKEN AND VEGGIE MIX

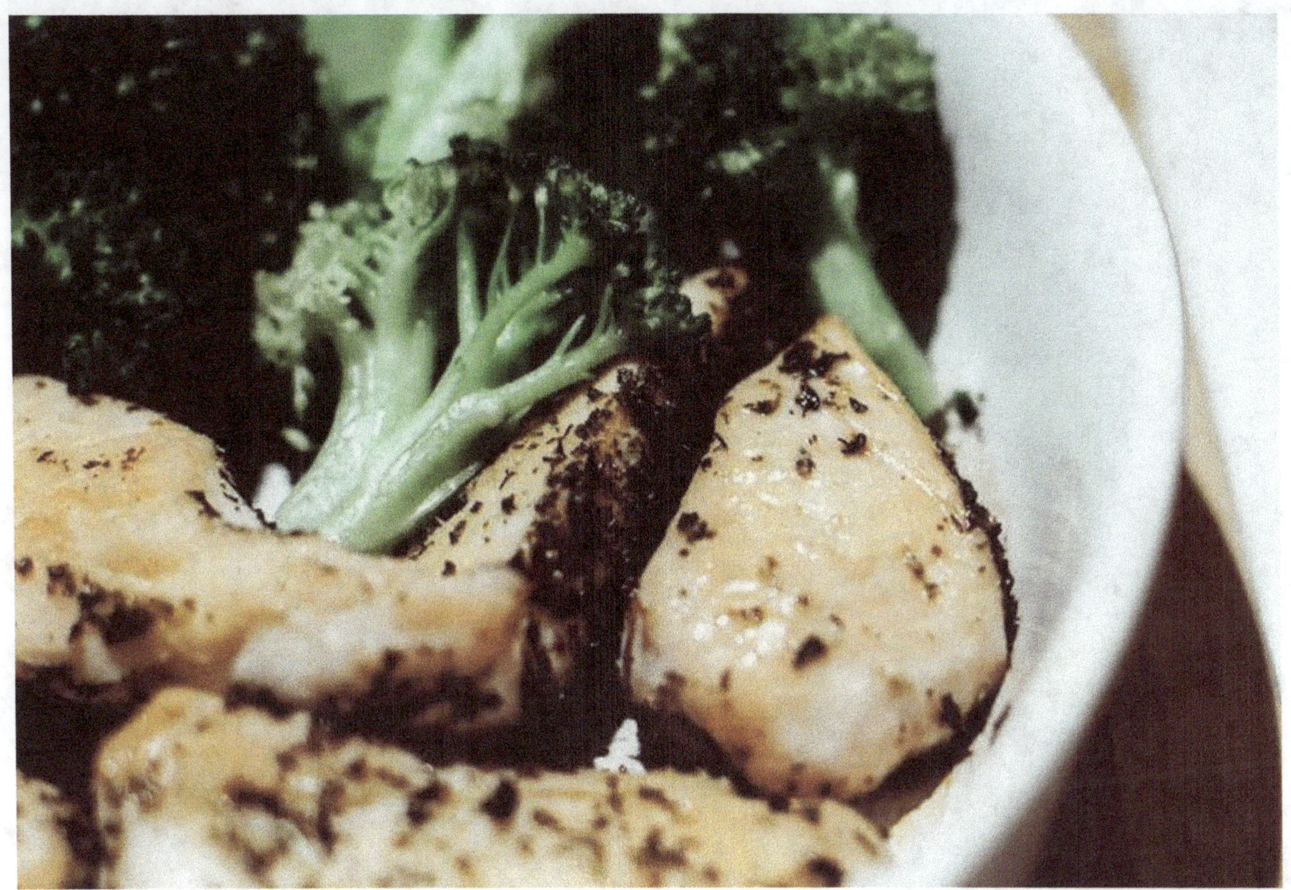

225 calories

What You'll Need:

- 4 oz raw chicken breast, cut into bite-sized pieces
- 1 cup mixed vegetables (like bell peppers, broccoli, and carrots)
- 1 tbsp soy sauce (low-sodium)
- 1 tsp olive oil

Directions:

- Preheat your air fryer to 375°F (190°C).
- In a bowl, toss the chicken pieces and mixed vegetables with the olive oil and soy sauce. Make sure everything is evenly coated.
- Place the chicken and vegetables in the air fryer basket in a single layer.
- Cook for 10-12 minutes, shaking the basket halfway through the cooking time, until the chicken is cooked through and the vegetables are tender.
- Serve warm.

BAKED TILAPIA

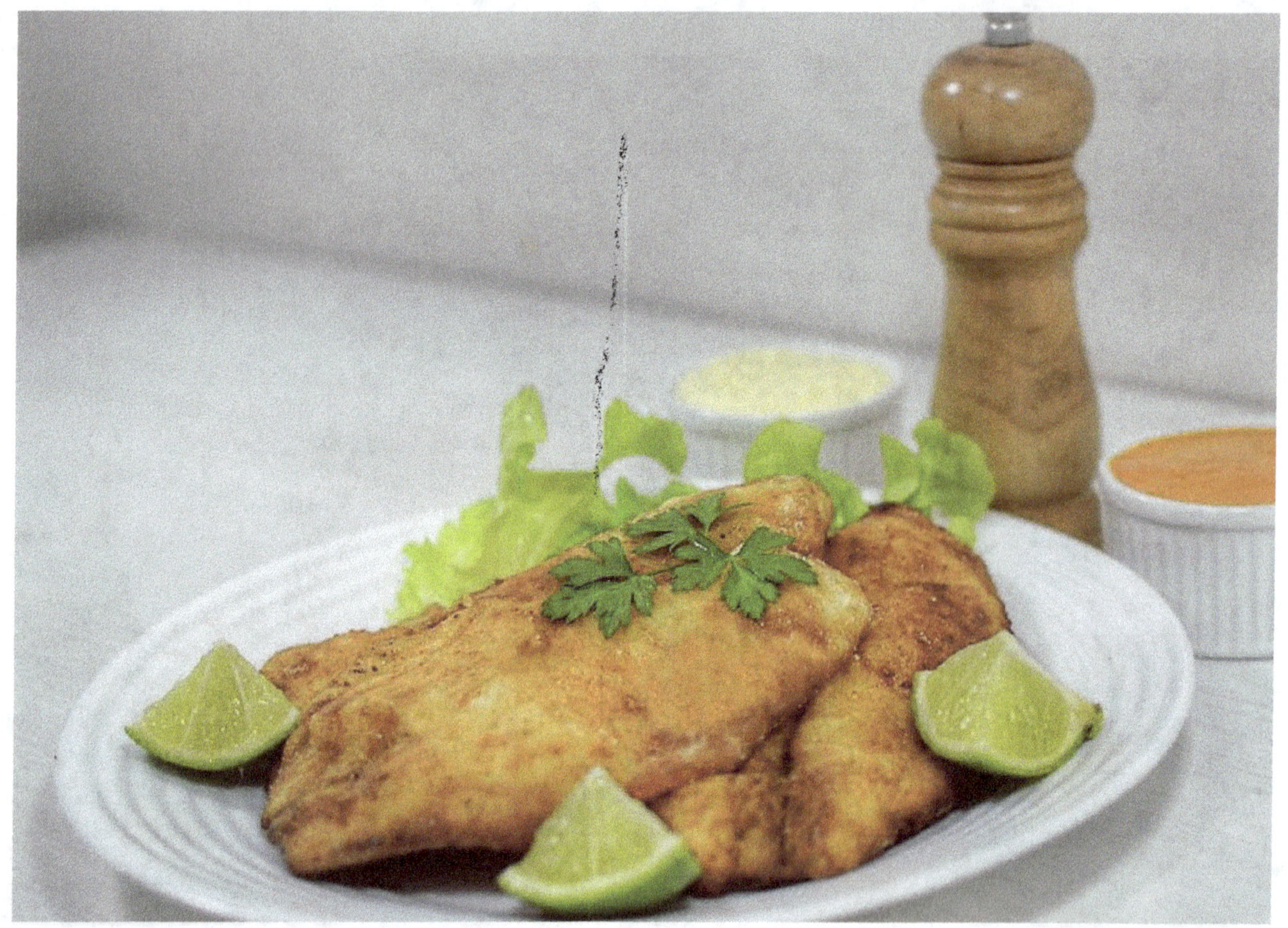

300 calories

What You'll Need:

- 4 oz tilapia fillet
- 1 lemon, sliced
- 1 tsp paprika
- 1 tbsp olive oil

Directions:

- Preheat oven to 400°F (200°C).
- Place tilapia on a baking sheet.
- Drizzle with olive oil and season with paprika.
- Top with lemon slices and bake for 15–20 minutes

VEGETABLE PAELLA

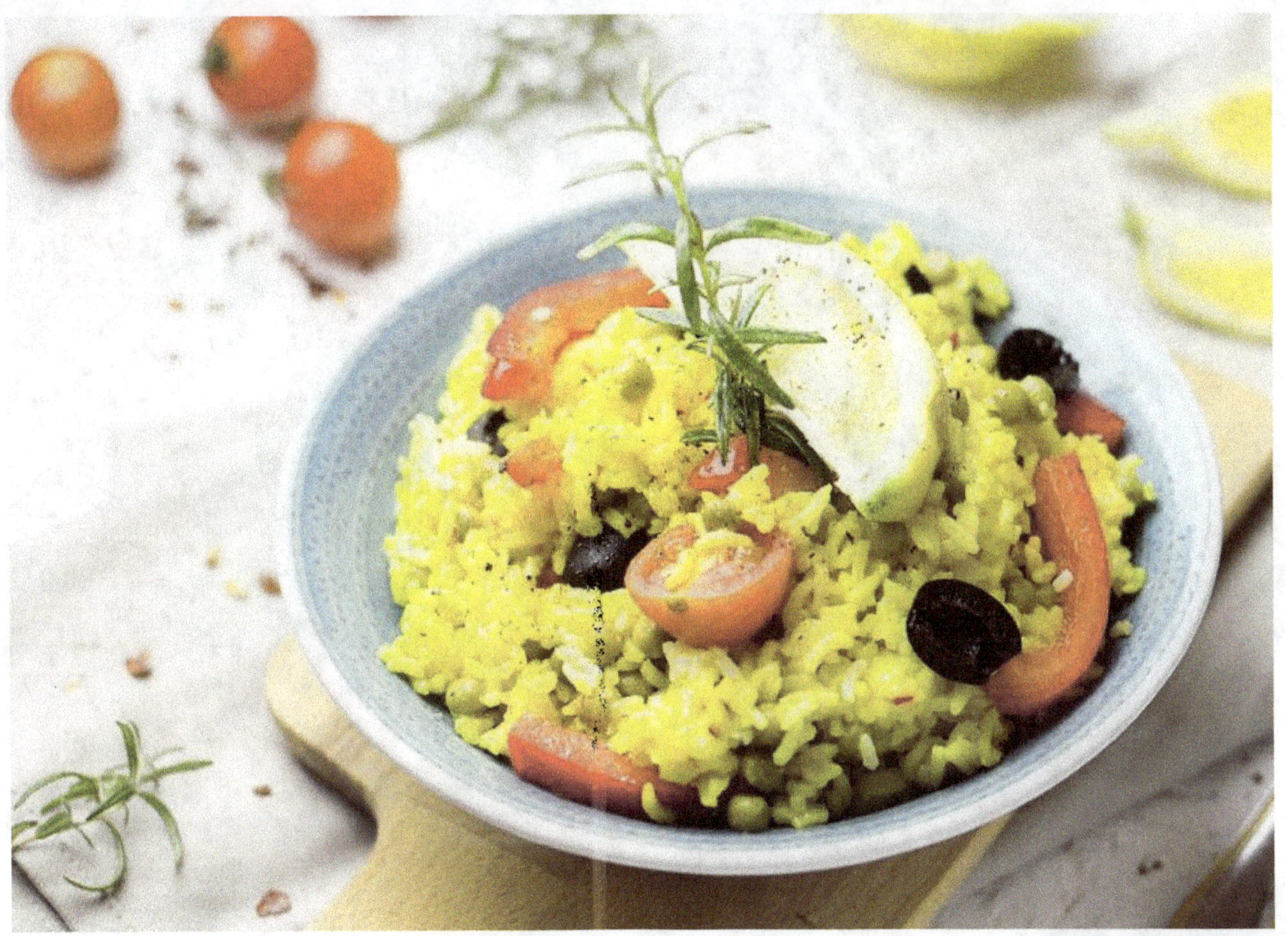

350 calories

What You'll Need:

- 1 cup rice
- 1 cup mixed vegetables (bell peppers, peas, tomatoes)
- 1 cup vegetable broth
- 1 tsp saffron

Directions:

- Sauté vegetables in a pan until tender.
- Add rice, vegetable broth, and saffron.
- Simmer until rice is cooked and liquid is absorbed.

TURKEY STUFFED PEPPERS

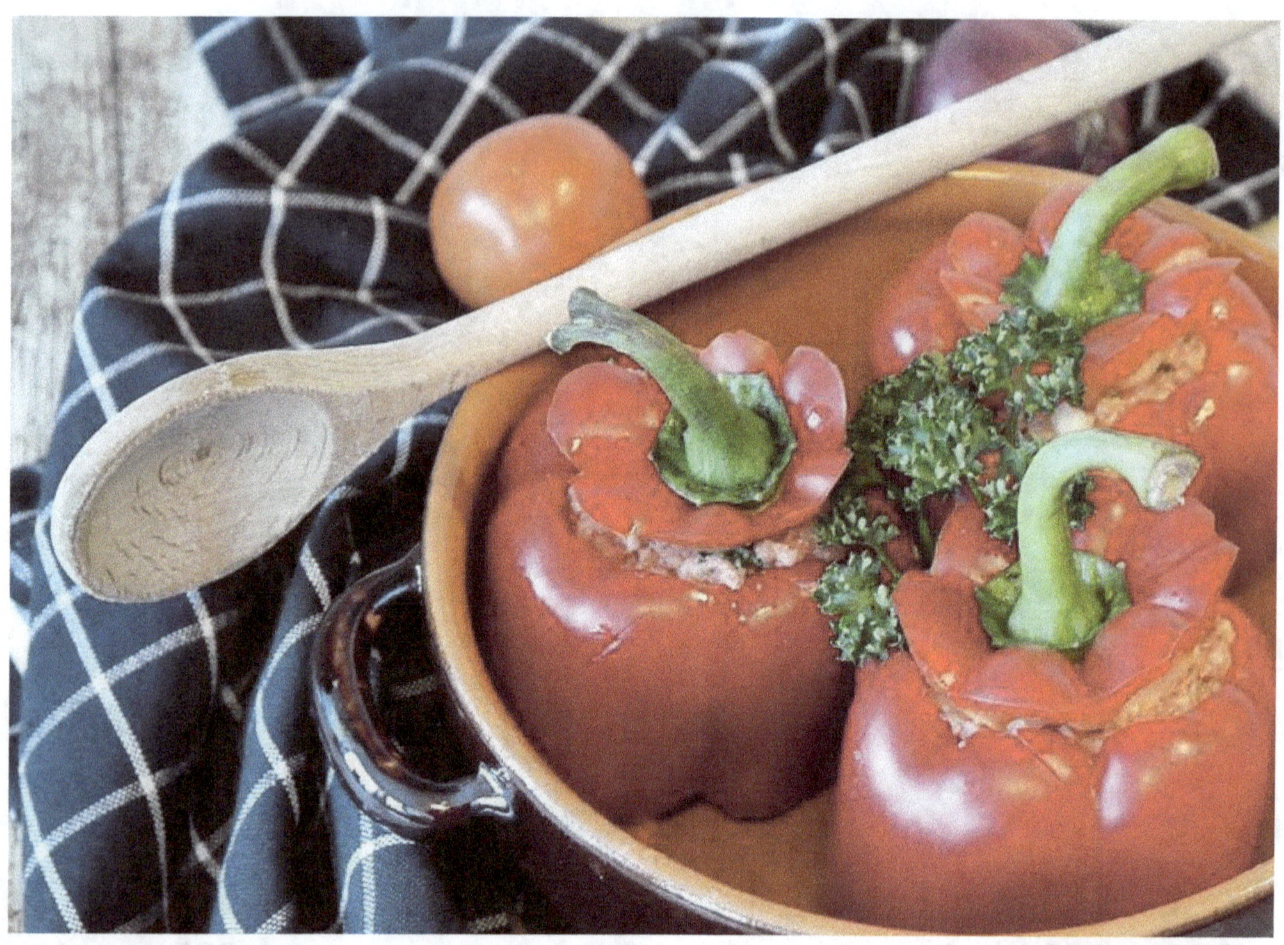

350 calories

What You'll Need:

- 2 bell peppers
- 1 cup cooked ground turkey
- ¼ cup cooked rice
- ½ cup tomato sauce

Directions:

- Preheat oven to 375°F (190°C).
- Mix ground turkey with rice and tomato sauce.
- Stuff bell peppers with the mixture.
- Bake for 30–35 minutes.

CAULIFLOWER FRIED RICE

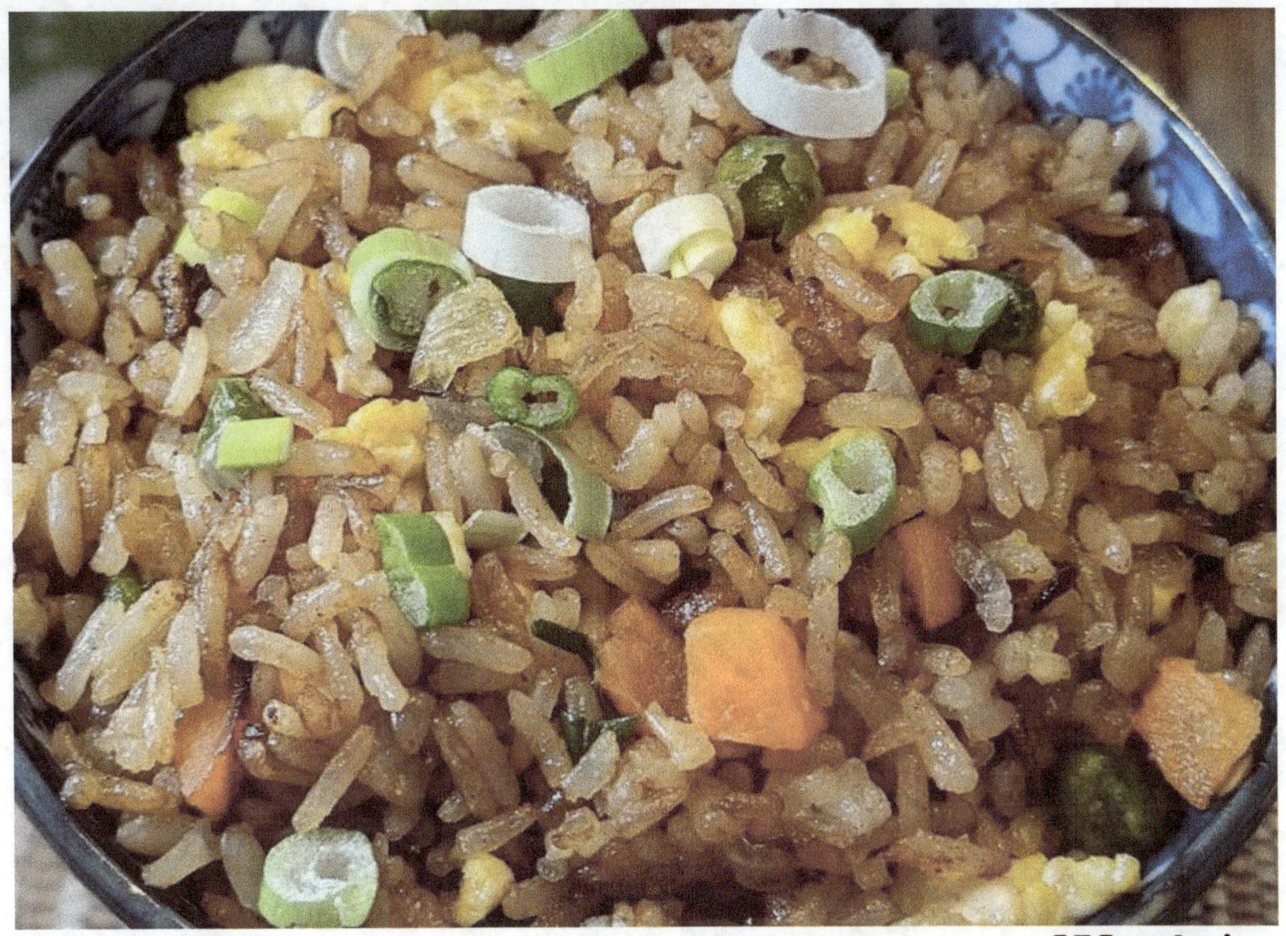

250 calories

What You'll Need:

- 2 cups cauliflower rice
- 1 cup mixed vegetables
- 2 eggs
- 2 tbsp soy sauce

Directions:

- Sauté vegetables in a pan until tender.
- Add cauliflower rice and cook until tender.
- Push vegetables to one side and scramble eggs on the other.
- Combine and stir in soy sauce before serving.

BBQ CHICKEN

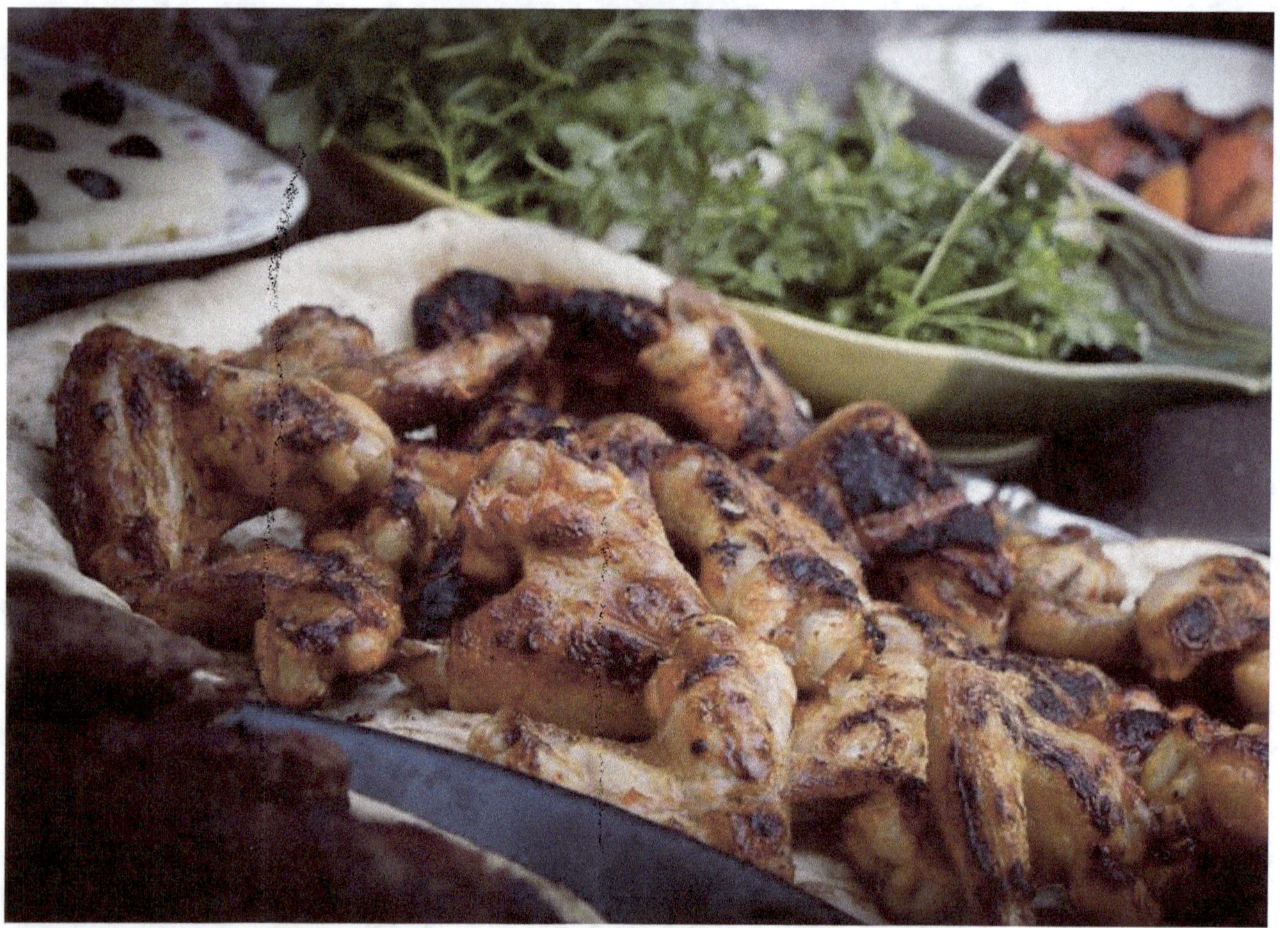

400 calories

What You'll Need:

- 4 oz chicken breast
- ¼ cup BBQ sauce
- 1 tbsp olive oil

Directions:

- Preheat grill to medium–high heat.
- Brush chicken with BBQ sauce and olive oil.
- Grill for 6–8 minutes per side.

MUSHROOM RISOTTO

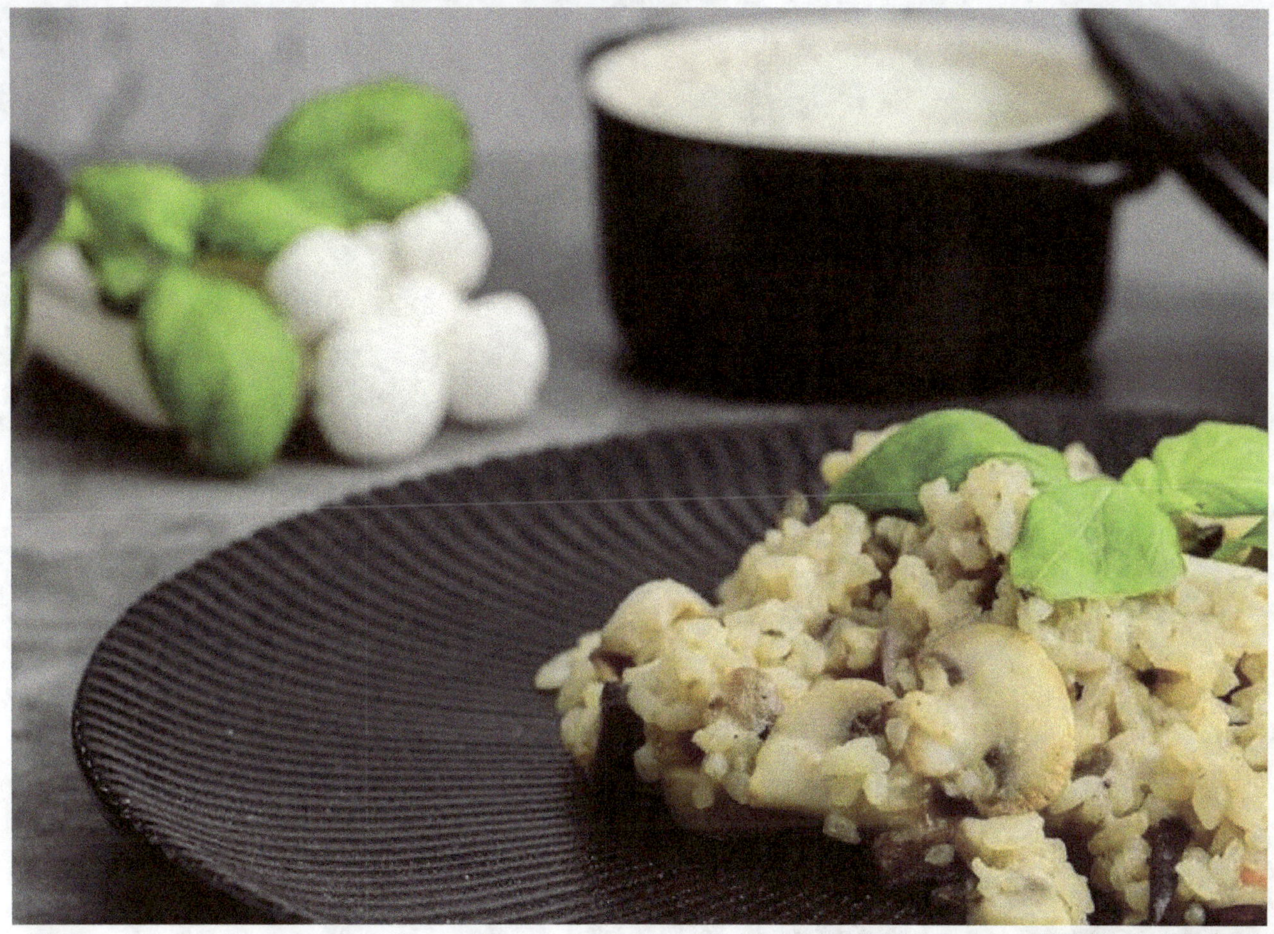

350 calories

What You'll Need:

- 1 cup Arborio rice
- 1 cup mushrooms, sliced
- 1 cup vegetable broth
- 1 tbsp olive oil
- ¼ cup Parmesan cheese

Directions:

- Sauté mushrooms in olive oil until tender.
- Add Arborio rice and cook for 2 minutes.
- Gradually add vegetable broth, stirring constantly until rice is cooked.
- Stir in Parmesan cheese before serving

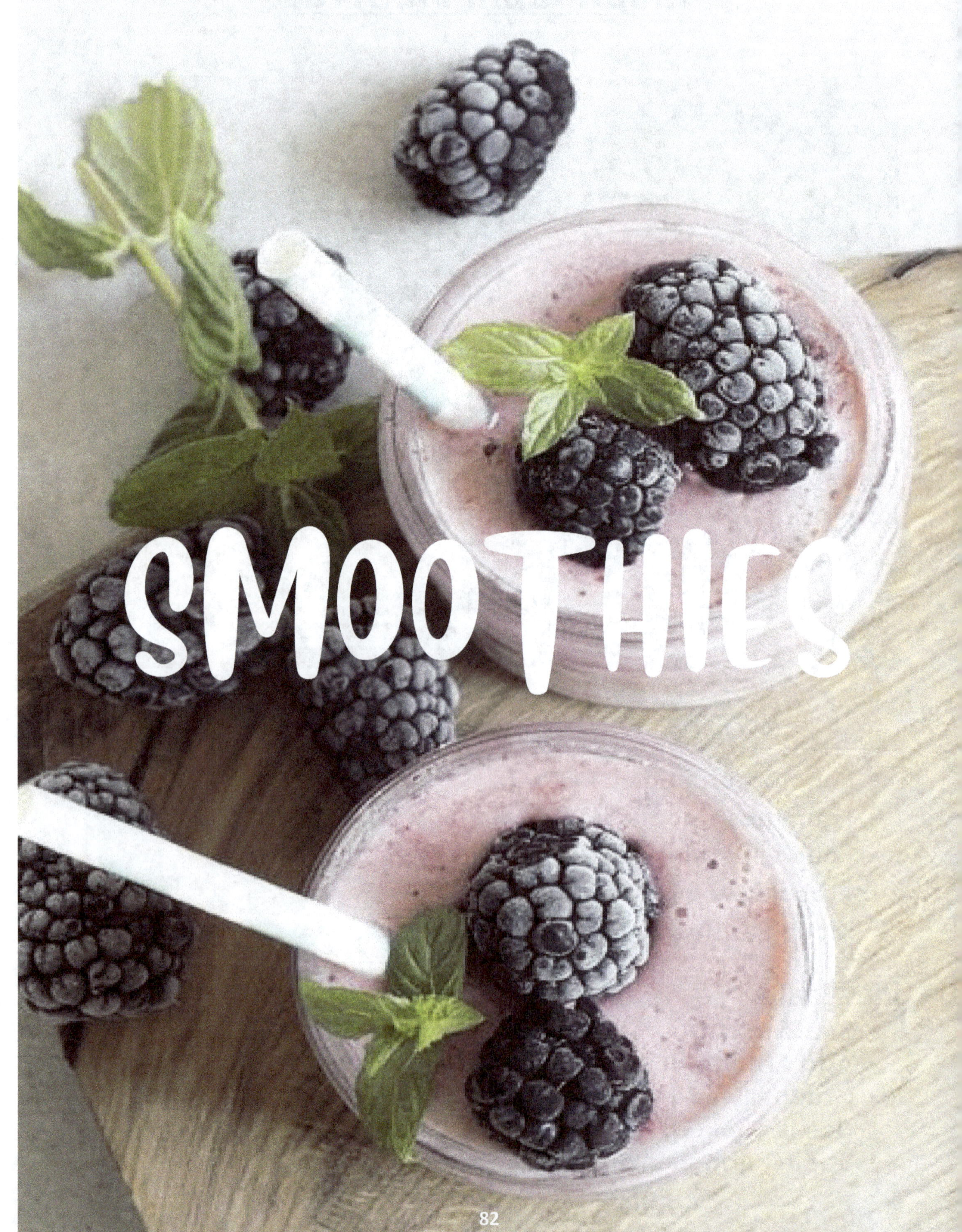

SMOOTHIES

BERRY BANANA SMOOTHIE

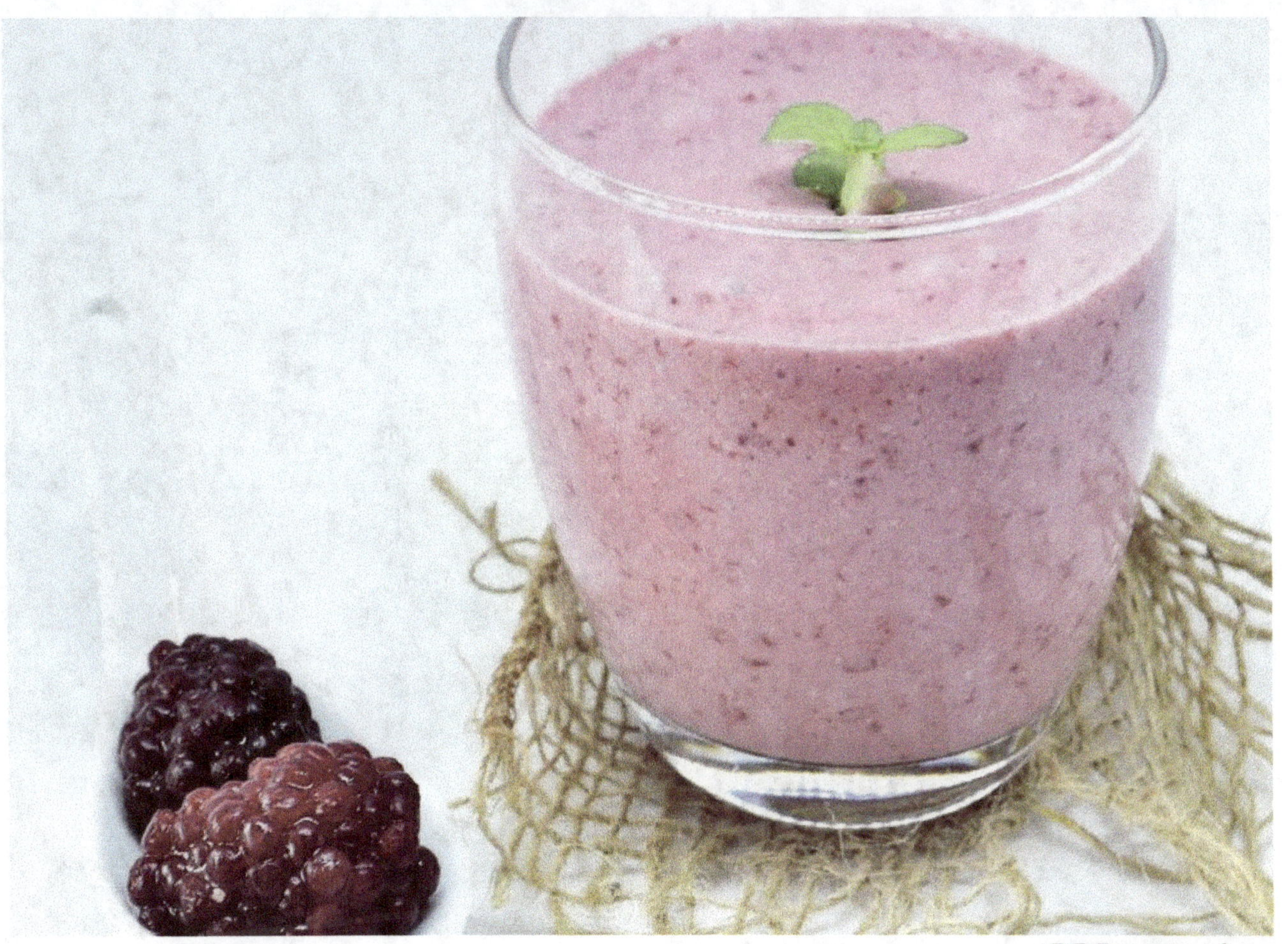

200 calories

What You'll Need:

- 1 banana
- ½ cup mixed berries (strawberries, blueberries, raspberries)
- 1 cup almond milk
- 1 tbsp honey

Directions:

- Blend all Ingredients until smooth.
- Pour into a glass and serve.

GREEN DETOX SMOOTHIE

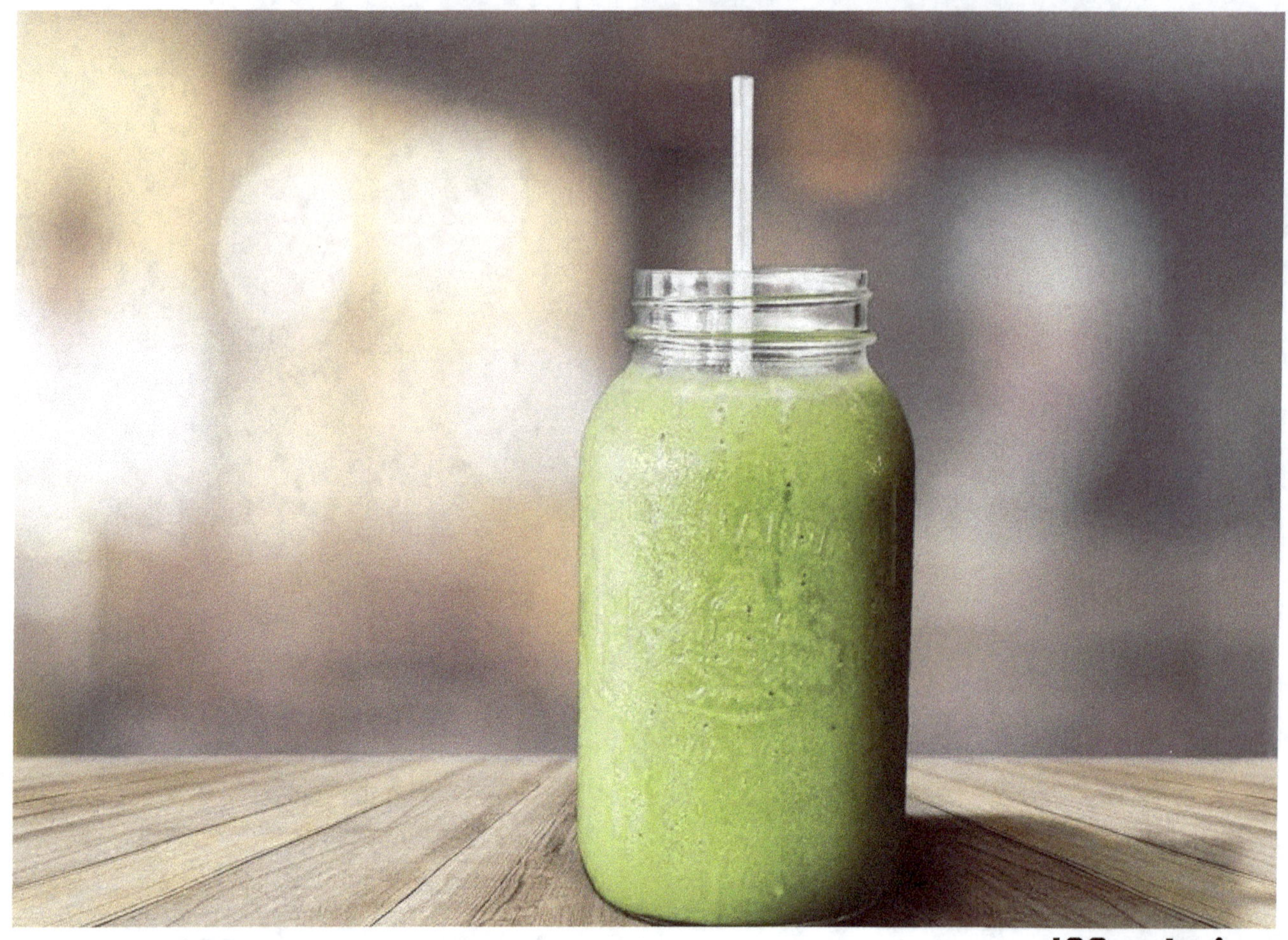

180 calories

What You'll Need:

- 1 cup spinach
- 1 green apple, cored
- ½ cucumber
- 1 tbsp lemon juice
- 1 cup water

Directions:

- Blend all Ingredients until smooth.
- Pour into a glass and serve.

MANGO PINEAPPLE SMOOTHIE

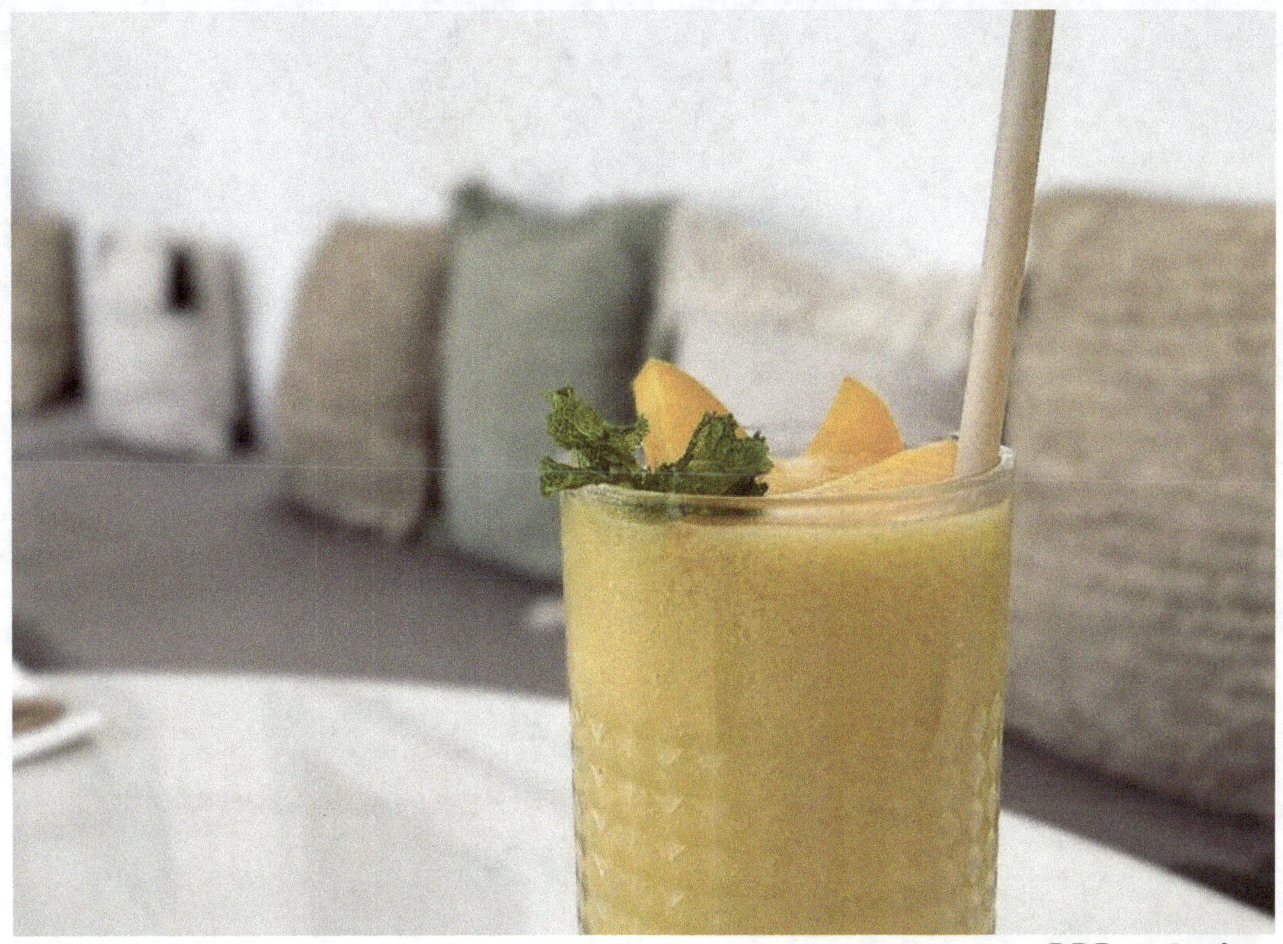

220 calories

What You'll Need:

- 1 cup mango chunks
- 1 cup pineapple chunks
- 1 cup coconut water
- 1 tbsp lime juice

Directions:

- Blend all Ingredients until smooth.
- Pour into a glass and serve.

STRAWBERRY OAT SMOOTHIE

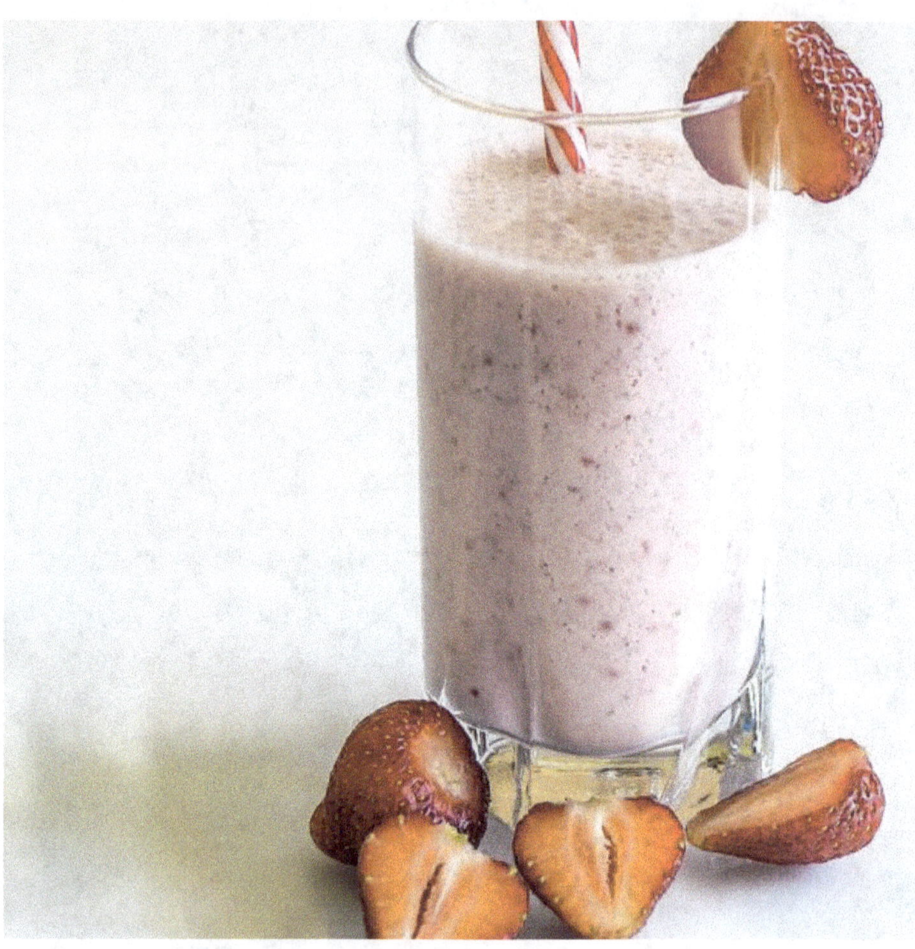

250 calories

What You'll Need:

- 1 cup strawberries
- ½ cup rolled oats
- 1 cup almond milk
- 1 tbsp chia seeds

Directions:

- Blend all Ingredients until smooth.
- Pour into a glass and serve.

PEANUT BUTTER BANANA SMOOTHIE

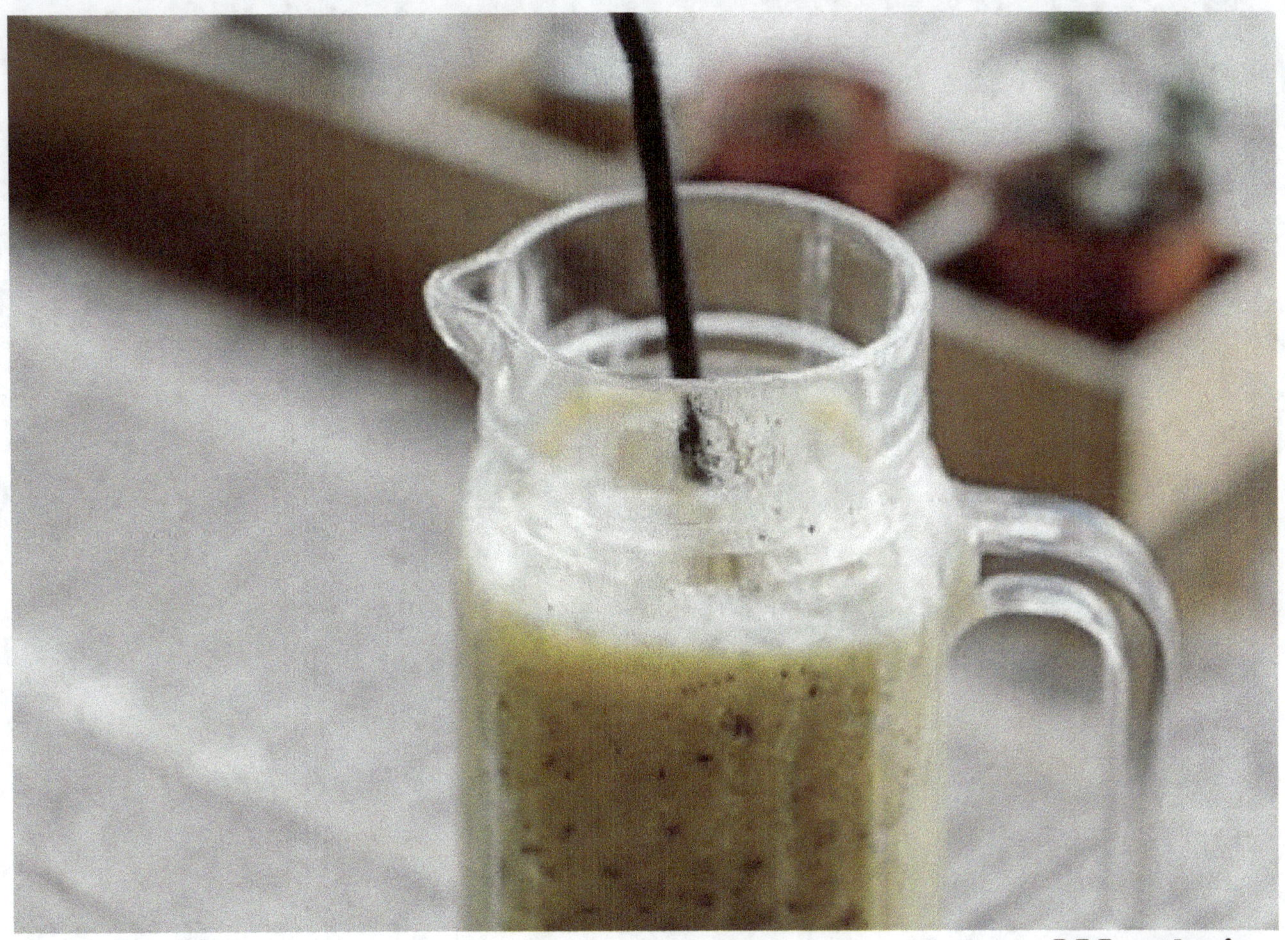

300 calories

What You'll Need:

- 1 banana
- 2 tbsp peanut butter
- 1 cup milk
- 1 tbsp honey

Directions:

- Blend all Ingredients until smooth.
- Pour into a glass and serve.

AVOCADO SPINACH SMOOTHIE

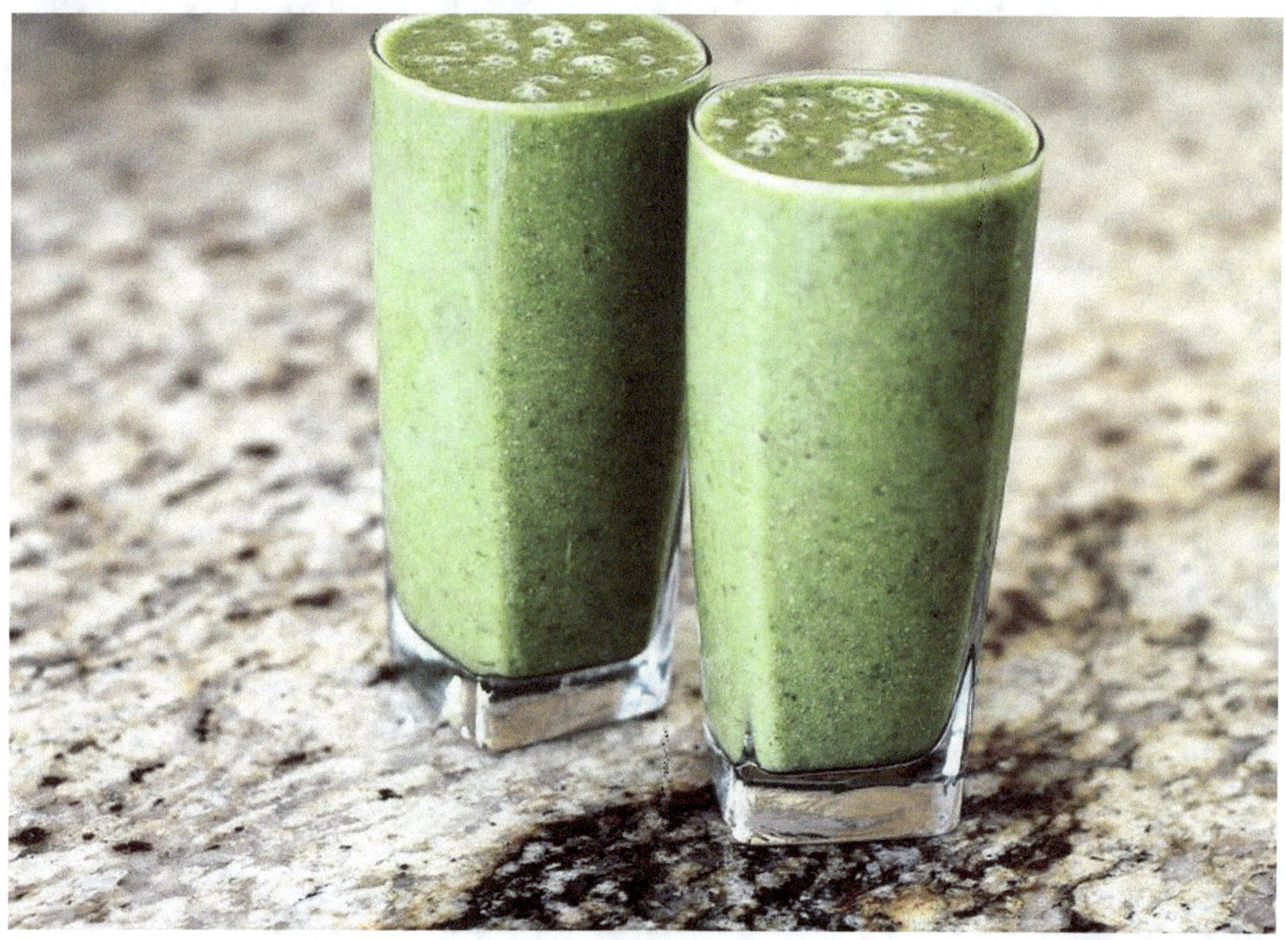

240 calories

What You'll Need:

- ½ avocado
- 1 cup spinach
- 1 banana
- 1 cup almond milk

Directions:

- Blend all Ingredients until smooth.
- Pour into a glass and serve.

BLUEBERRY ALMOND SMOOTHIE

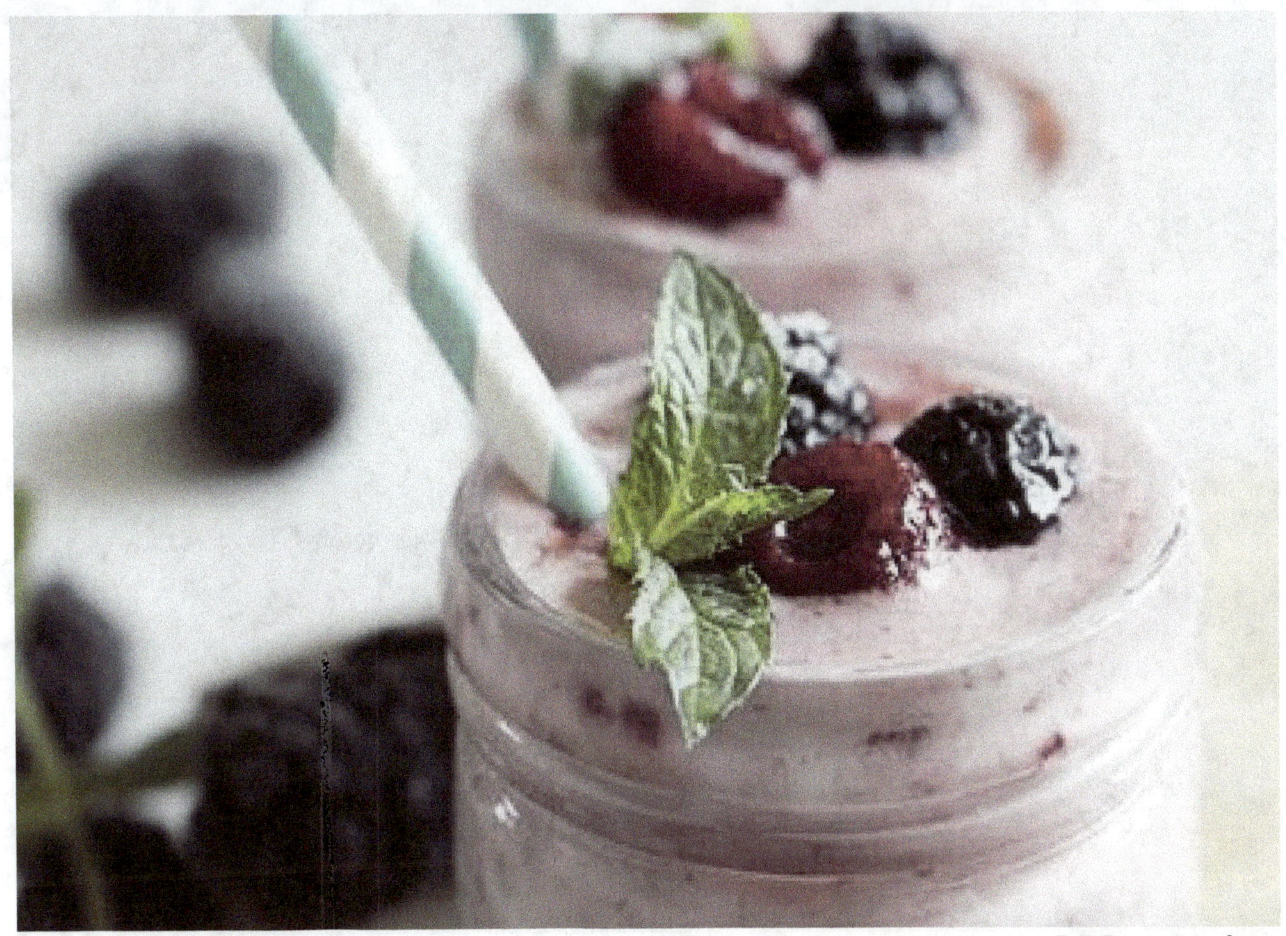

200 calories

What You'll Need:

- 1 cup blueberries
- 1 tbsp almond butter
- 1 cup almond milk
- 1 tsp honey

Directions:

- Blend all Ingredients until smooth.
- Pour into a glass and serve.

TROPICAL KALE SMOOTHIE

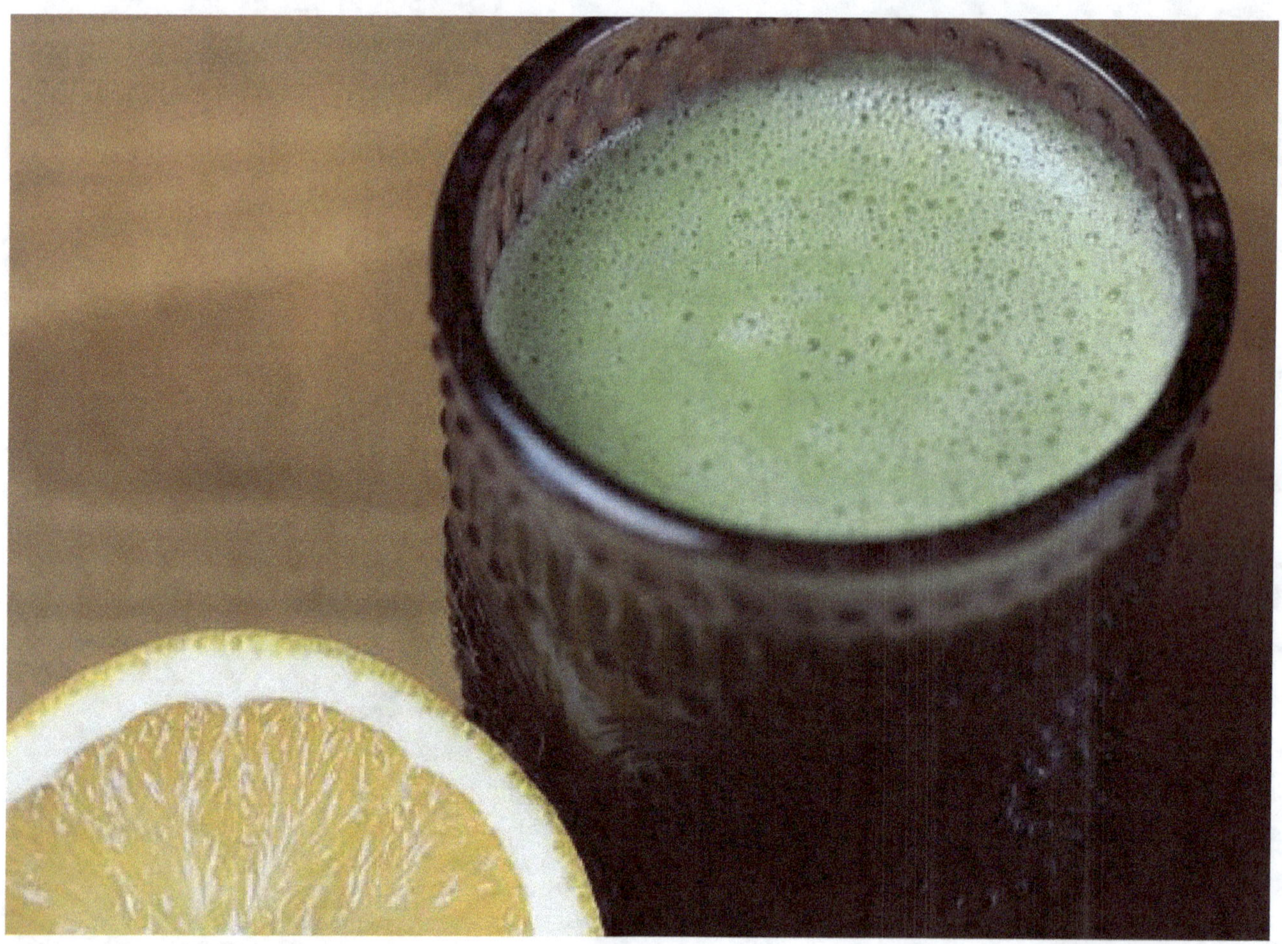

180 calories

What You'll Need:

- 1 cup kale
- 1 cup pineapple chunks
- 1 banana
- 1 cup coconut water

Directions:

- Blend all Ingredients until smooth.
- Pour into a glass and serve.

CHOCOLATE PROTEIN SMOOTHIE

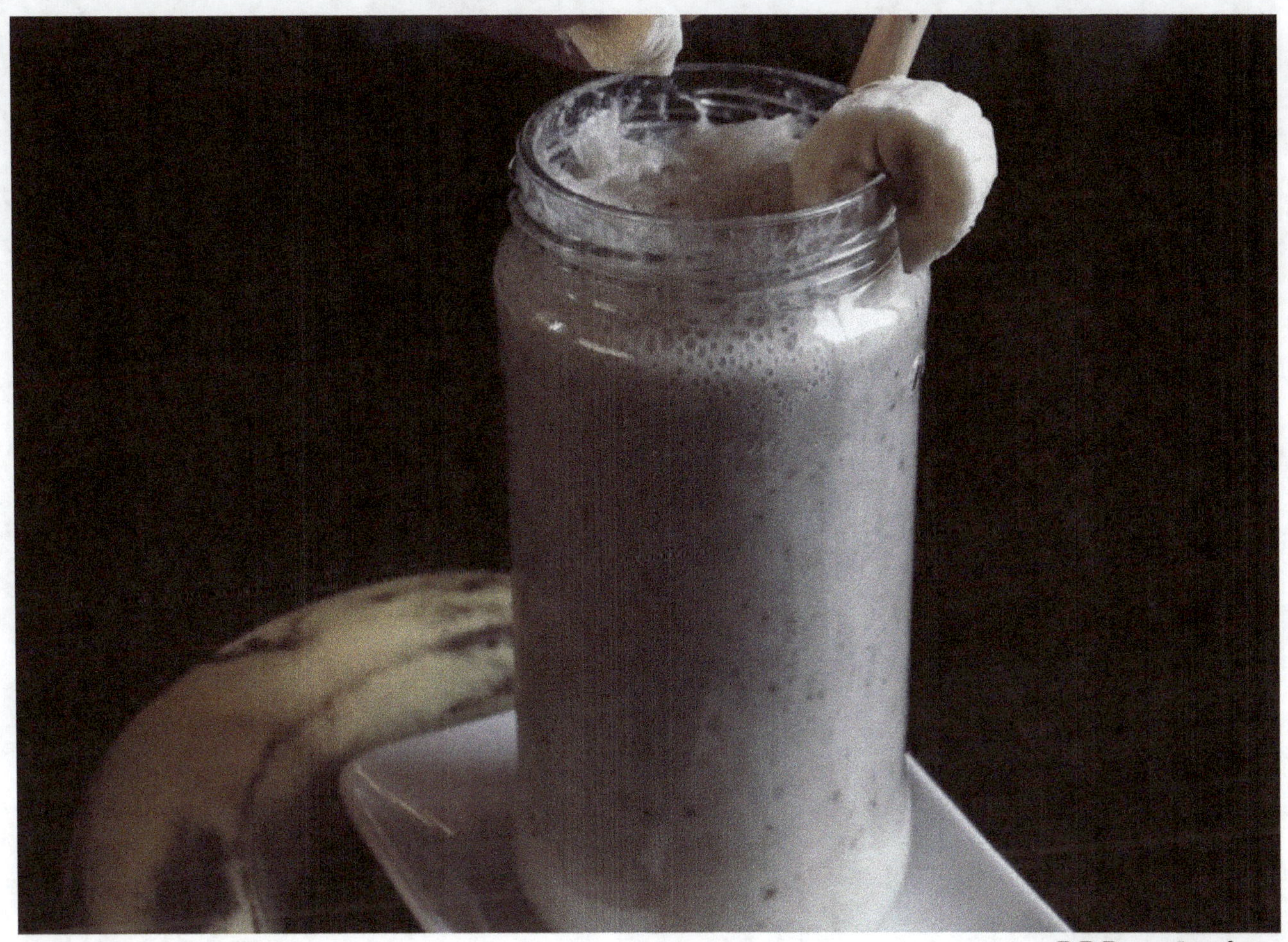

300 calories

What You'll Need:

- 1 scoop chocolate protein powder
- 1 banana
- 1 cup almond milk
- 1 tbsp peanut butter

Directions:

- Blend all Ingredients until smooth.
- Pour into a glass and serve.

COCONUT BERRY SMOOTHIE

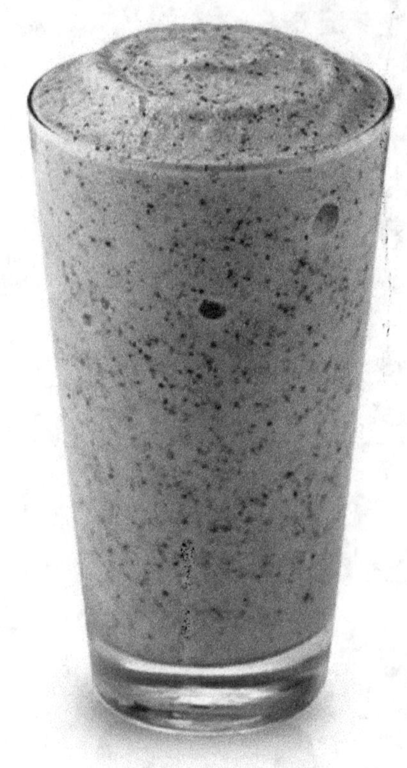

220 calories

<u>What You'll Need:</u>

- ½ cup mixed berries
- 1 cup coconut milk
- 1 banana
- 1 tbsp honey

<u>Directions:</u>

- Blend all Ingredients until smooth.
- Pour into a glass and serve.

ORANGE CARROT SMOOTHIE

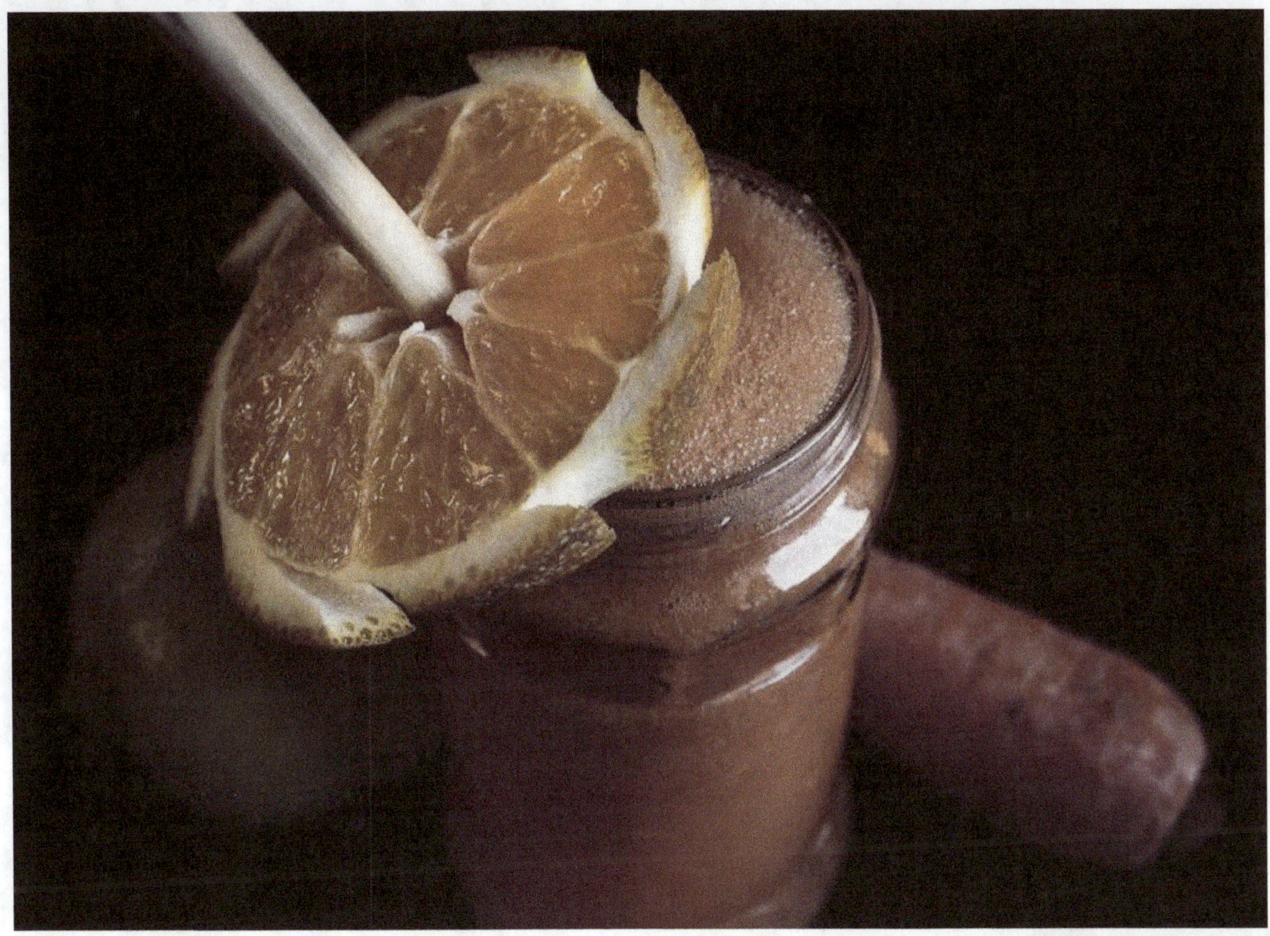

180 calories

What You'll Need:

- 1 cup carrot juice
- 1 orange, peeled
- ½ cup pineapple chunks
- 1 tsp ginger

Directions:

- Blend all Ingredients until smooth.
- Pour into a glass and serve.

KIWI SPINACH SMOOTHIE

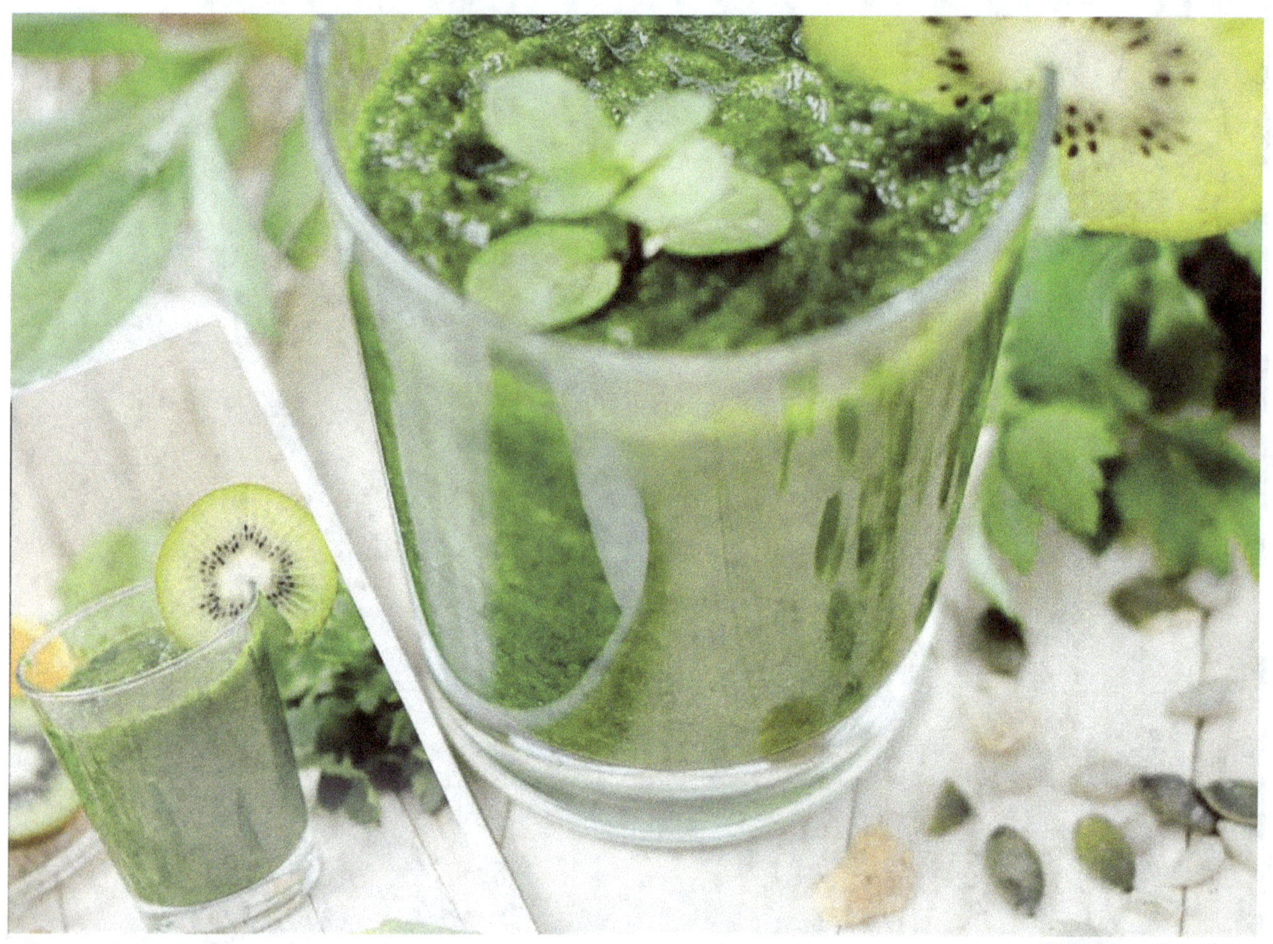

200 calories

What You'll Need:

- 2 kiwis, peeled
- 1 cup spinach
- 1 banana
- 1 cup almond milk

Directions:

- Blend all Ingredients until smooth.
- Pour into a glass and serve.

PEACH GINGER SMOOTHIE

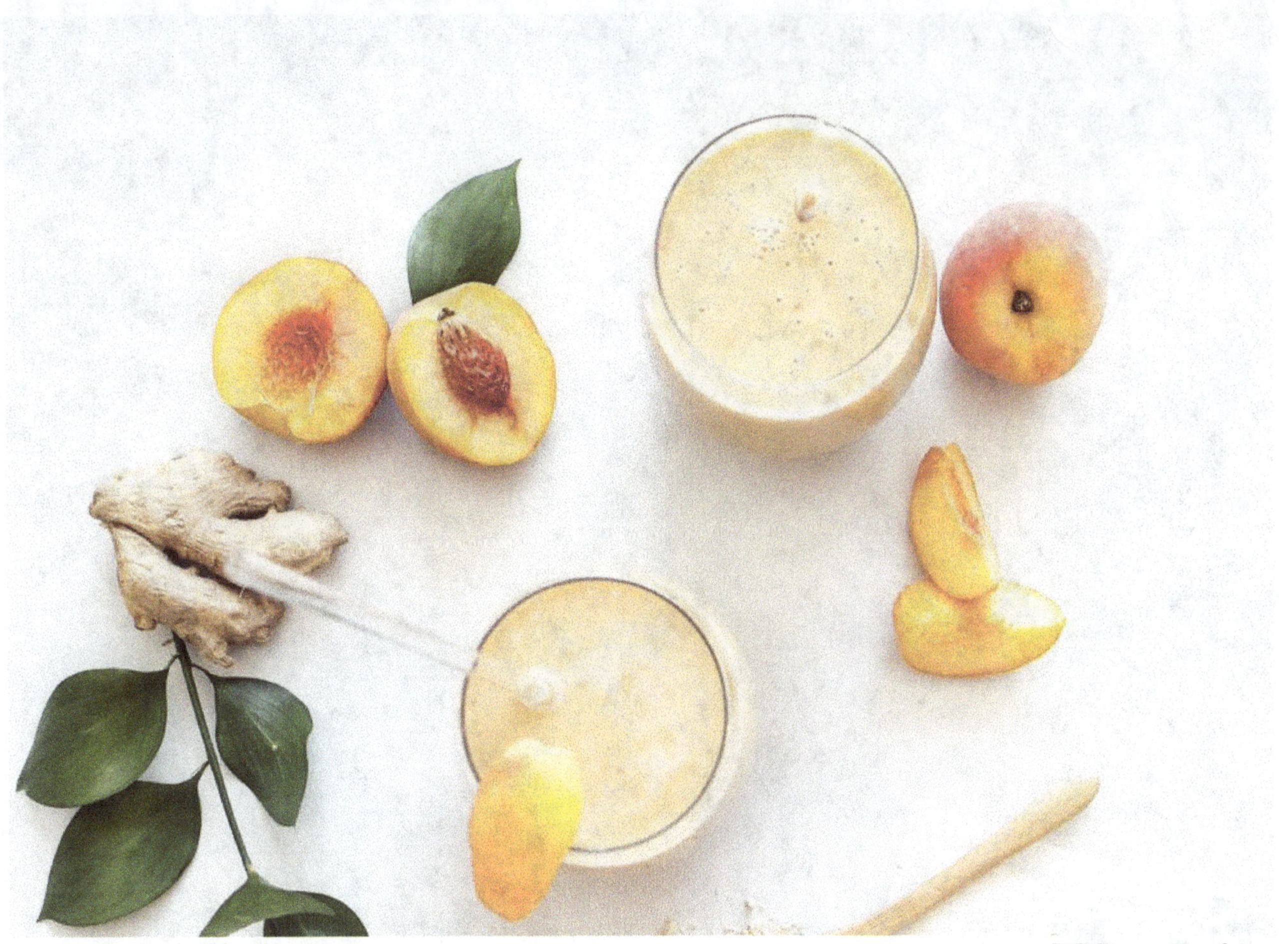

220 calories

What You'll Need:

- 1 cup peaches
- 1 tsp fresh ginger
- 1 cup almond milk
- 1 tbsp honey

Directions:

- Blend all Ingredients until smooth.
- Pour into a glass and serve.

APPLE CINNAMON SMOOTHIE

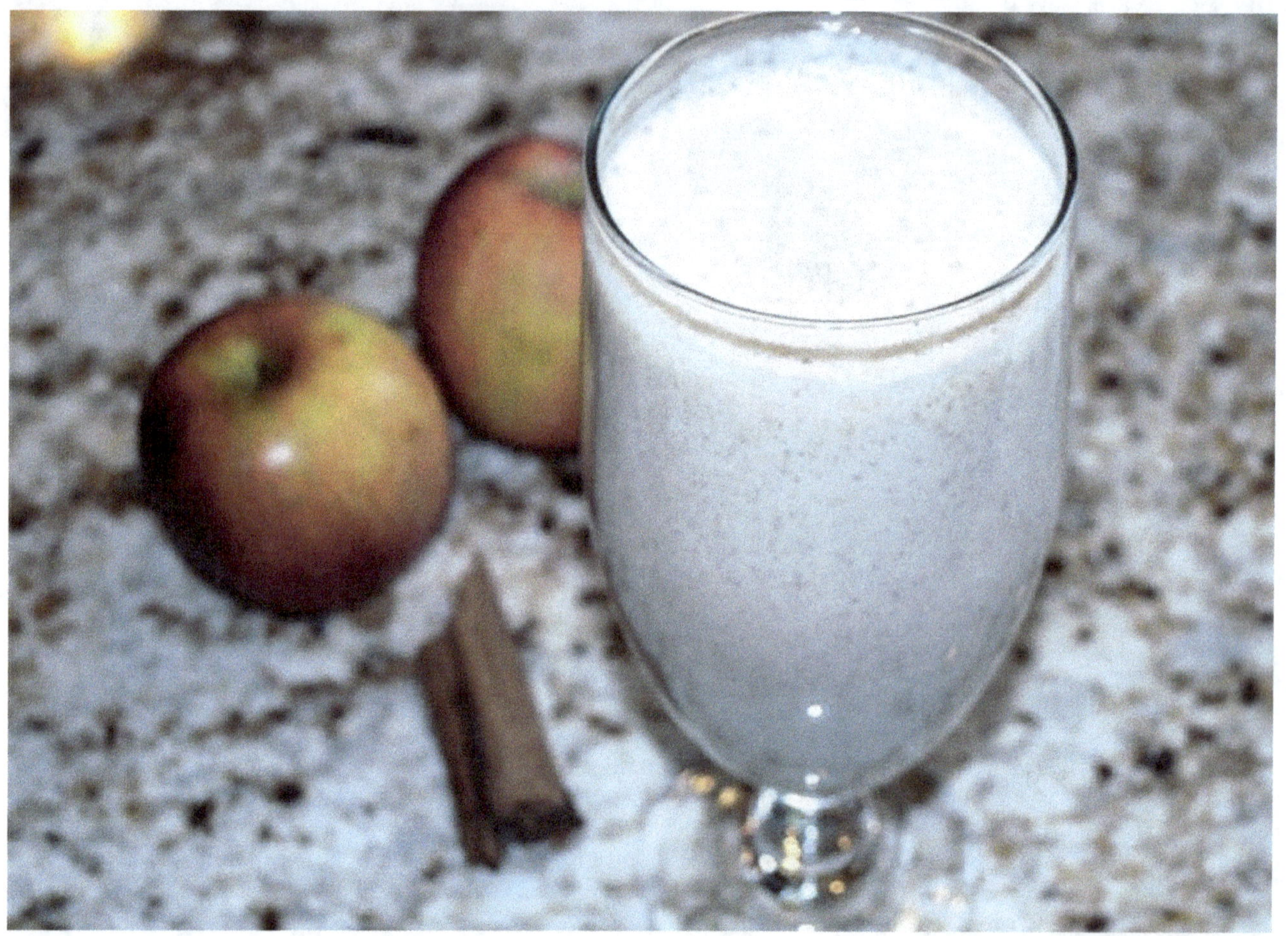

250 calories

What You'll Need:

- 1 apple, cored
- 1 tsp cinnamon
- 1 cup almond milk
- 1 tbsp honey

Directions:

- Blend all Ingredients until smooth.
- Pour into a glass and serve.

RASPBERRY CHIA SMOOTHIE

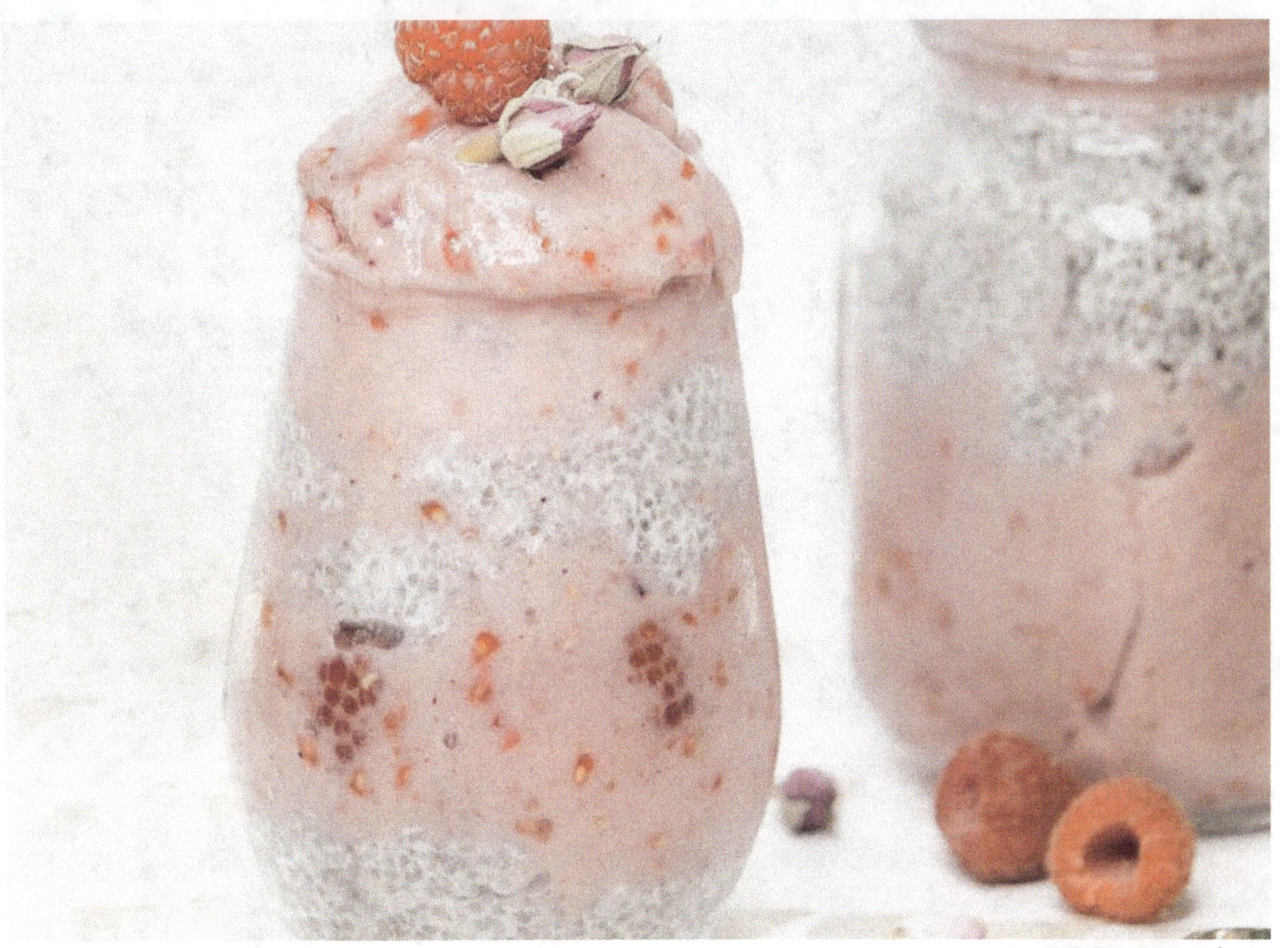

200 calories

<u>**What You'll Need:**</u>

- 1 cup raspberries
- 1 tbsp chia seeds
- 1 cup almond milk
- 1 tsp honey

<u>**Directions:**</u>

- Blend all Ingredients until smooth.
- Pour into a glass and serve.

PINEAPPLE COCONUT SMOOTHIE

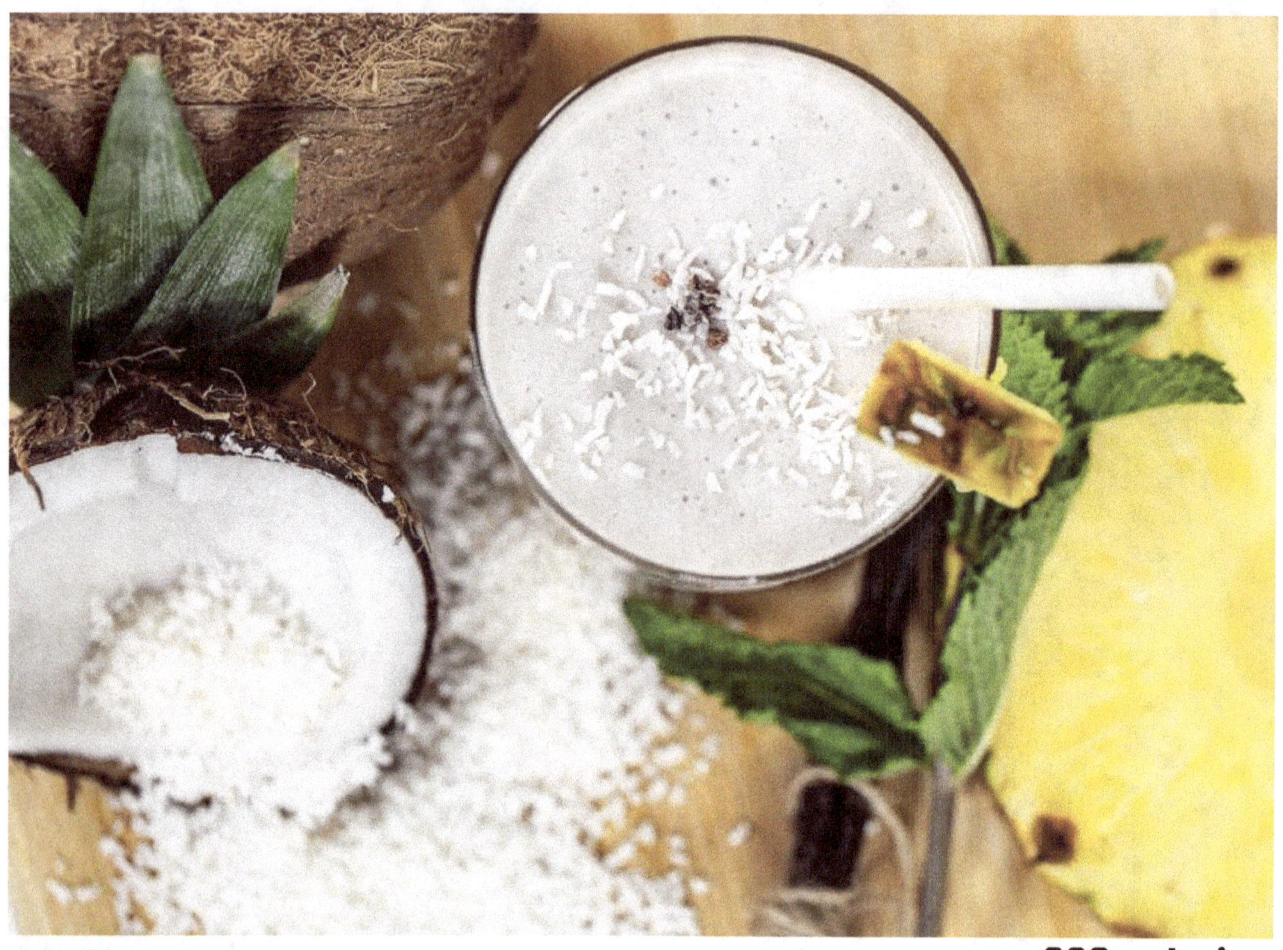

230 calories

<u>What You'll Need:</u>

- 1 cup pineapple chunks
- 1 cup coconut milk
- 1 banana
- 1 tbsp honey

<u>Directions:</u>

- Blend all Ingredients until smooth.
- Pour into a glass and serve.

CHERRY VANILLA SMOOTHIE

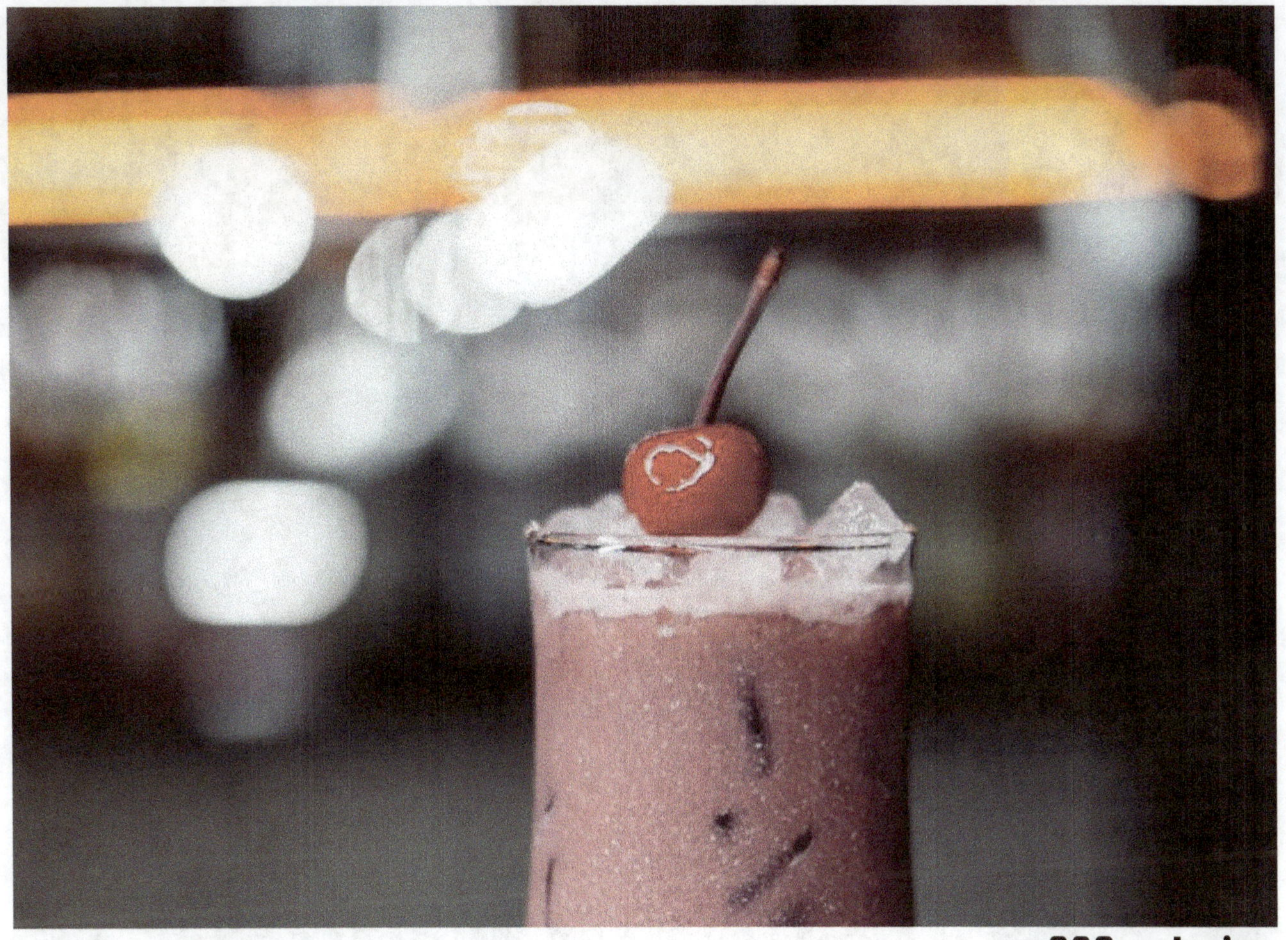

220 calories

What You'll Need:

- 1 cup cherries, pitted
- 1 tsp vanilla extract
- 1 cup almond milk
- 1 tbsp honey

Directions:

- Blend all Ingredients until smooth.
- Pour into a glass and serve.

PUMPKIN SPICE SMOOTHIE

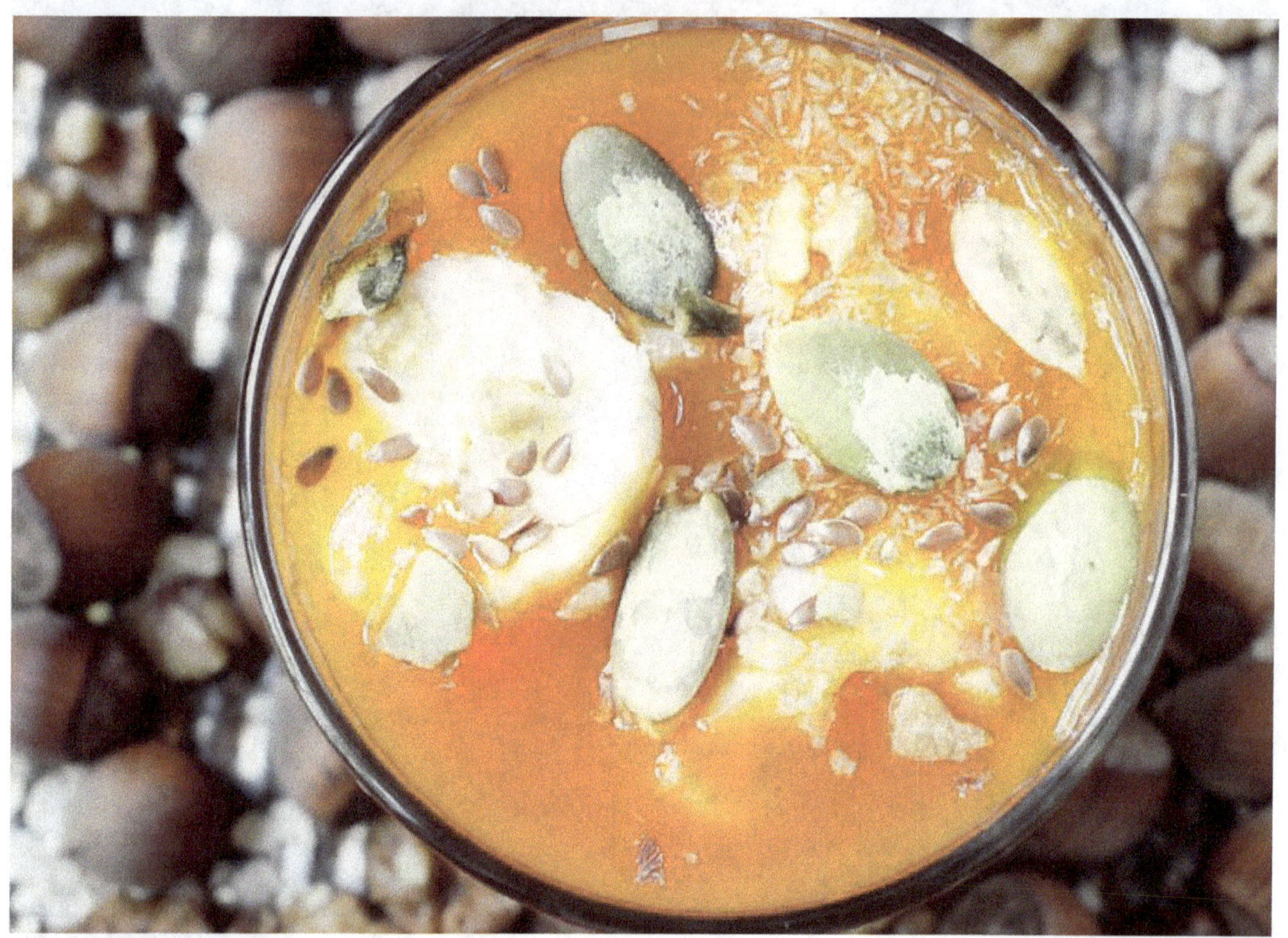

240 calories

What You'll Need:

- 1 cup pumpkin puree
- 1 banana
- 1 cup almond milk
- 1 tsp pumpkin spice

Directions:

- Blend all Ingredients until smooth.
- Pour into a glass and serve.

LEMON BLUEBERRY SMOOTHIE

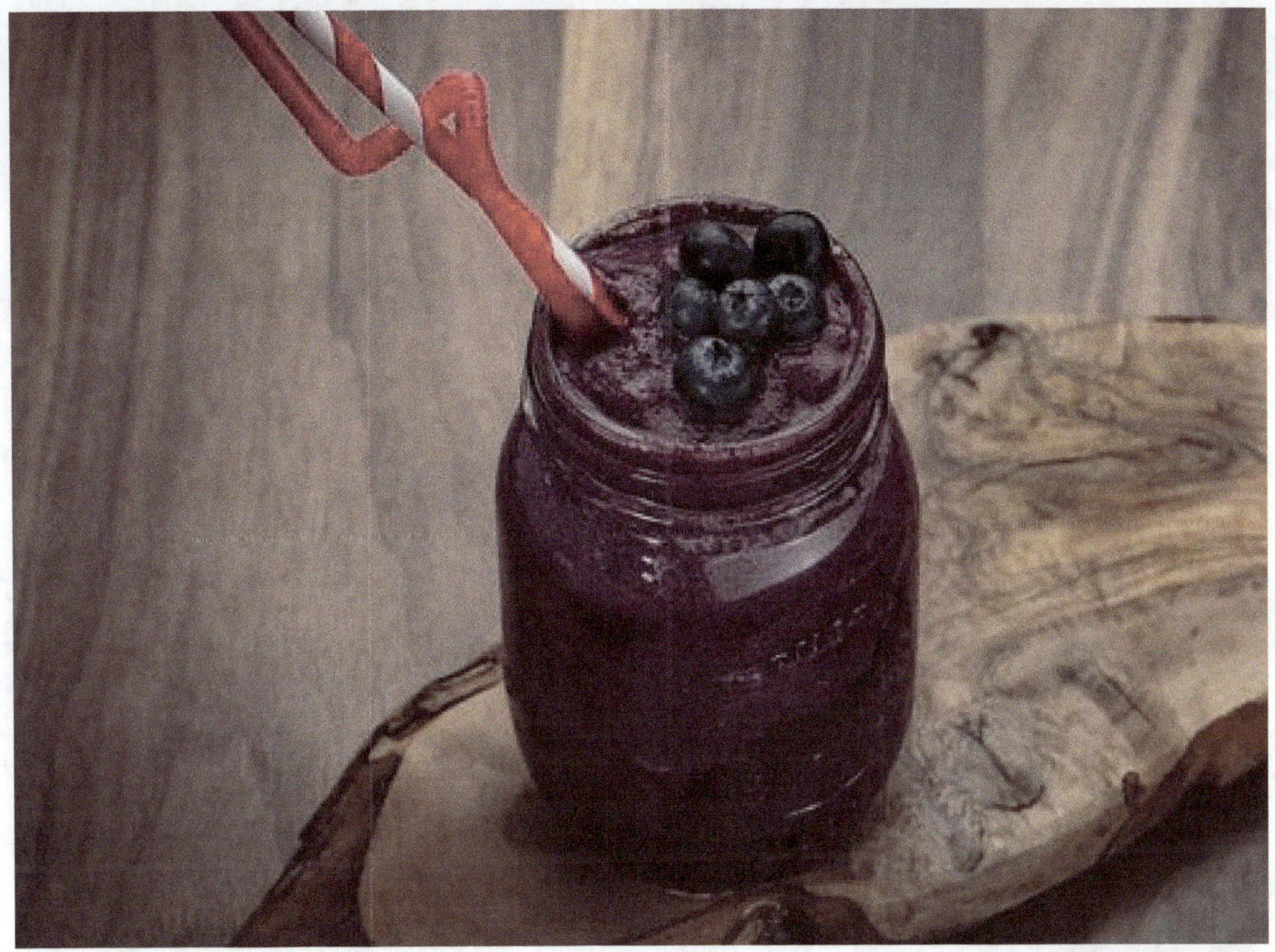

210 calories

What You'll Need:

- 1 cup blueberries
- 1 lemon, juiced
- 1 cup almond milk
- 1 tbsp honey

Directions:

- Blend all Ingredients until smooth.
- Pour into a glass and serve.

BANANA ALMOND SMOOTHIE

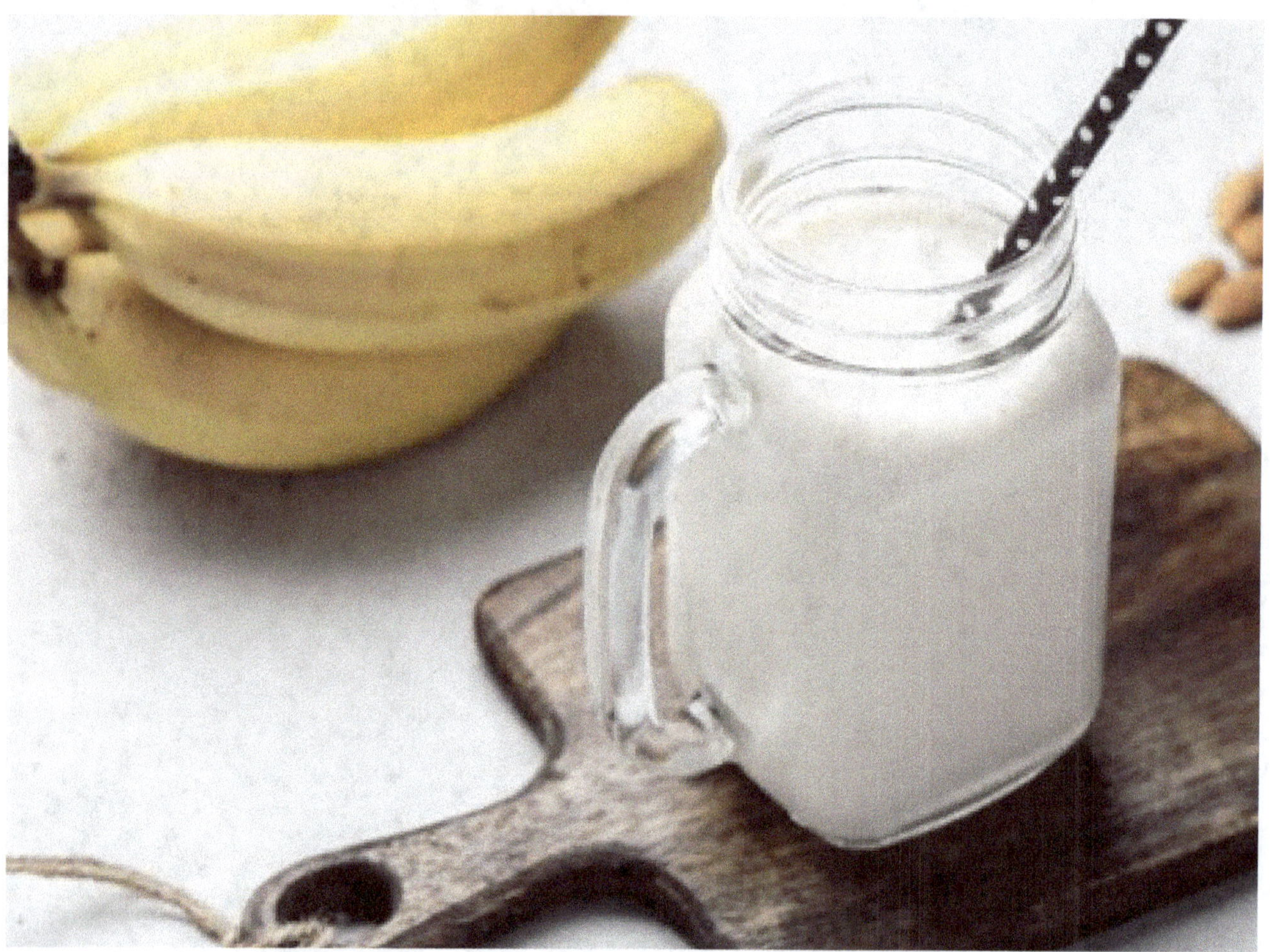

230 calories

What You'll Need:

- 1 banana
- 1 tbsp almond butter
- 1 cup almond milk
- 1 tsp honey

Directions:

- Blend all Ingredients until smooth.
- Pour into a glass and serve.

DESSERTS

CHIA SEED PUDDING

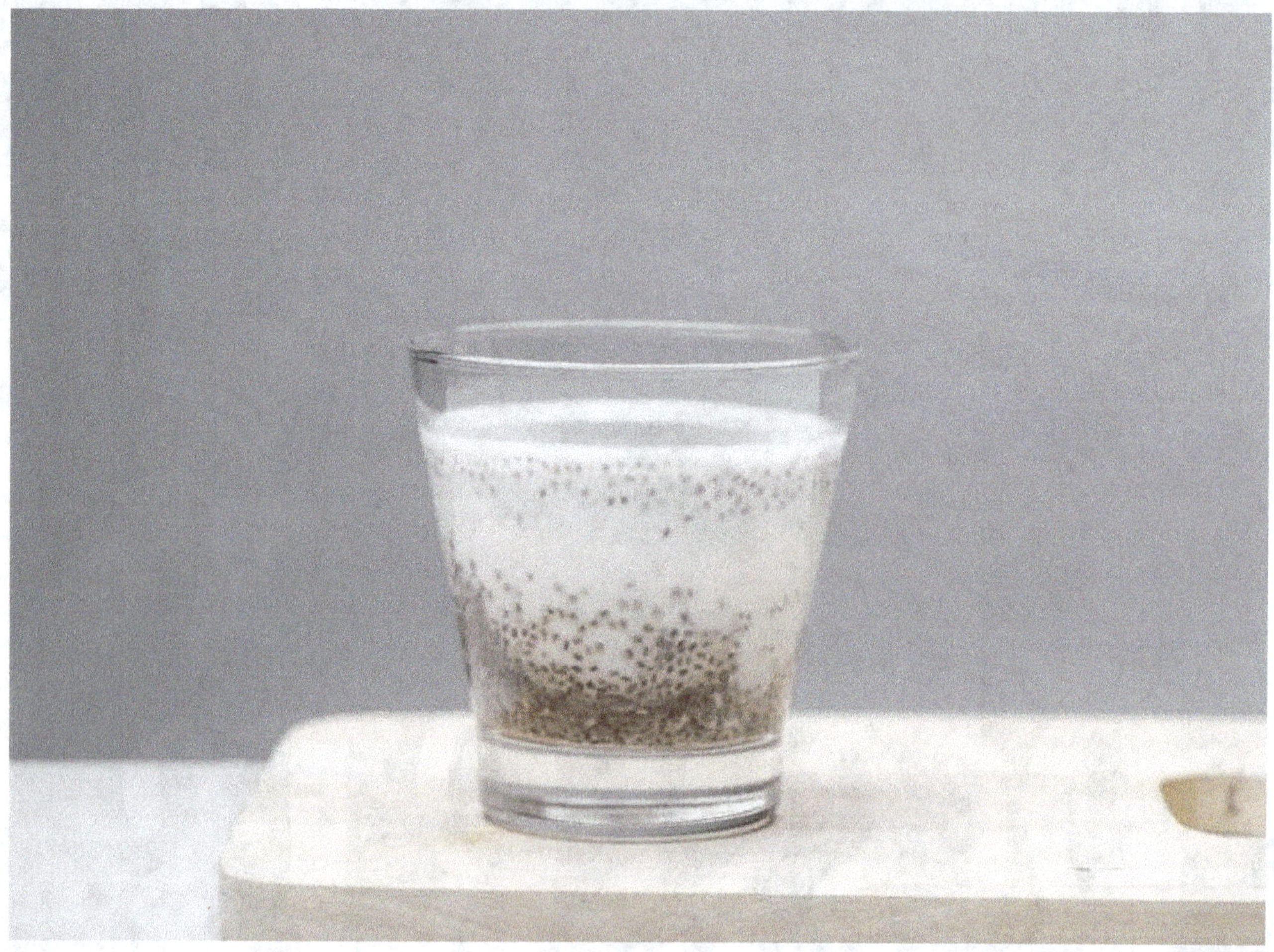

200 calories

What You'll Need:

- ¼ cup chia seeds
- 1 cup almond milk (or other milk)
- 1 tbsp honey or maple syrup
- ½ tsp vanilla extract

Directions:

- Mix chia seeds, almond milk, honey, and vanilla extract in a bowl.
- Refrigerate for at least 4 hours or overnight until thickened.
- Serve chilled.

FRUIT SORBET

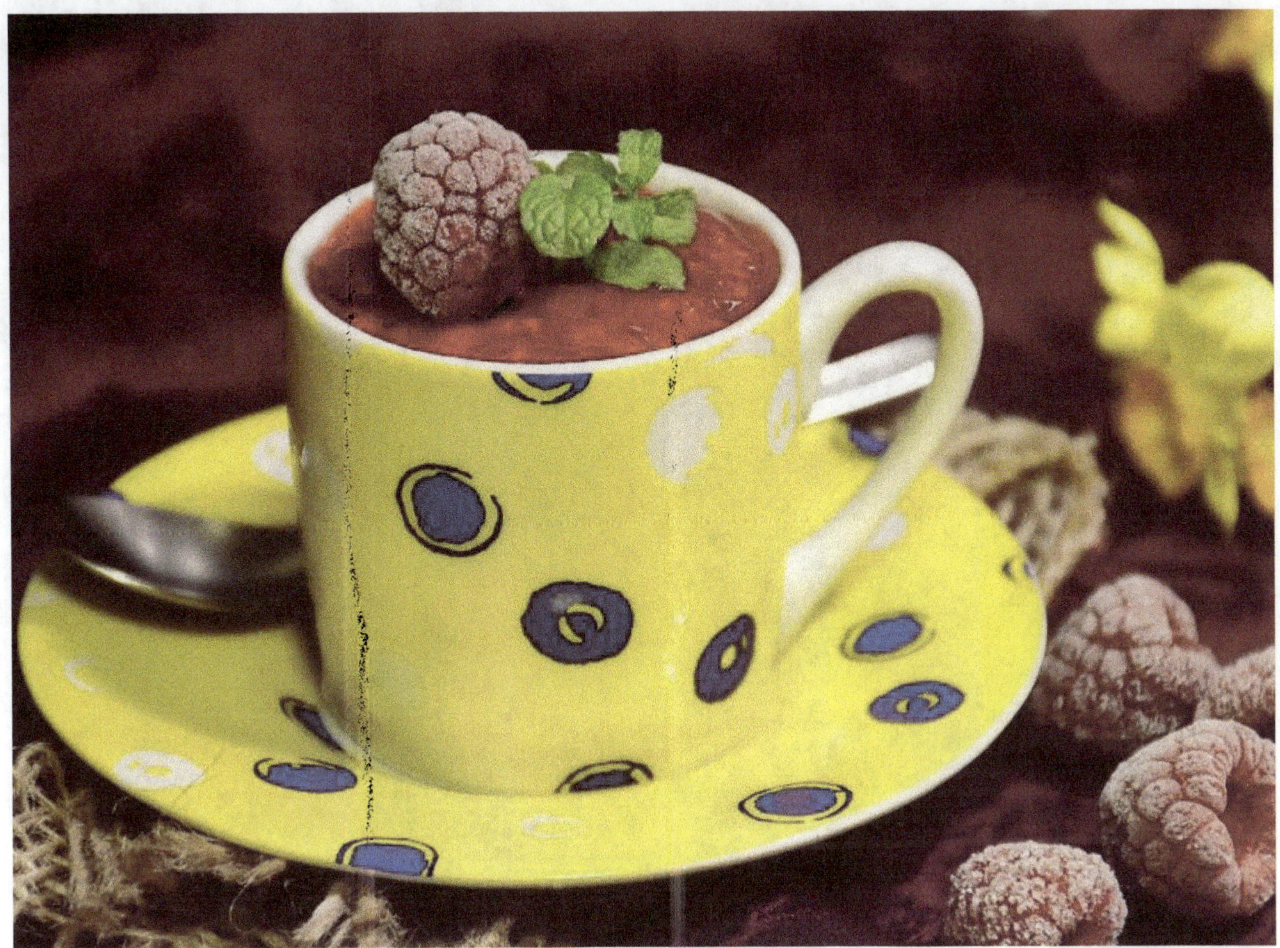

150 calories

What You'll Need:

- 1 cup fruit (such as mango, raspberry, or strawberry)
- 2 tbsp honey or agave syrup
- 1 tbsp lemon juice

Directions:

- Blend fruit, honey, and lemon juice until smooth.
- Pour into a container and freeze until firm.
- Scoop and serve.

DARK CHOCOLATE ALMON

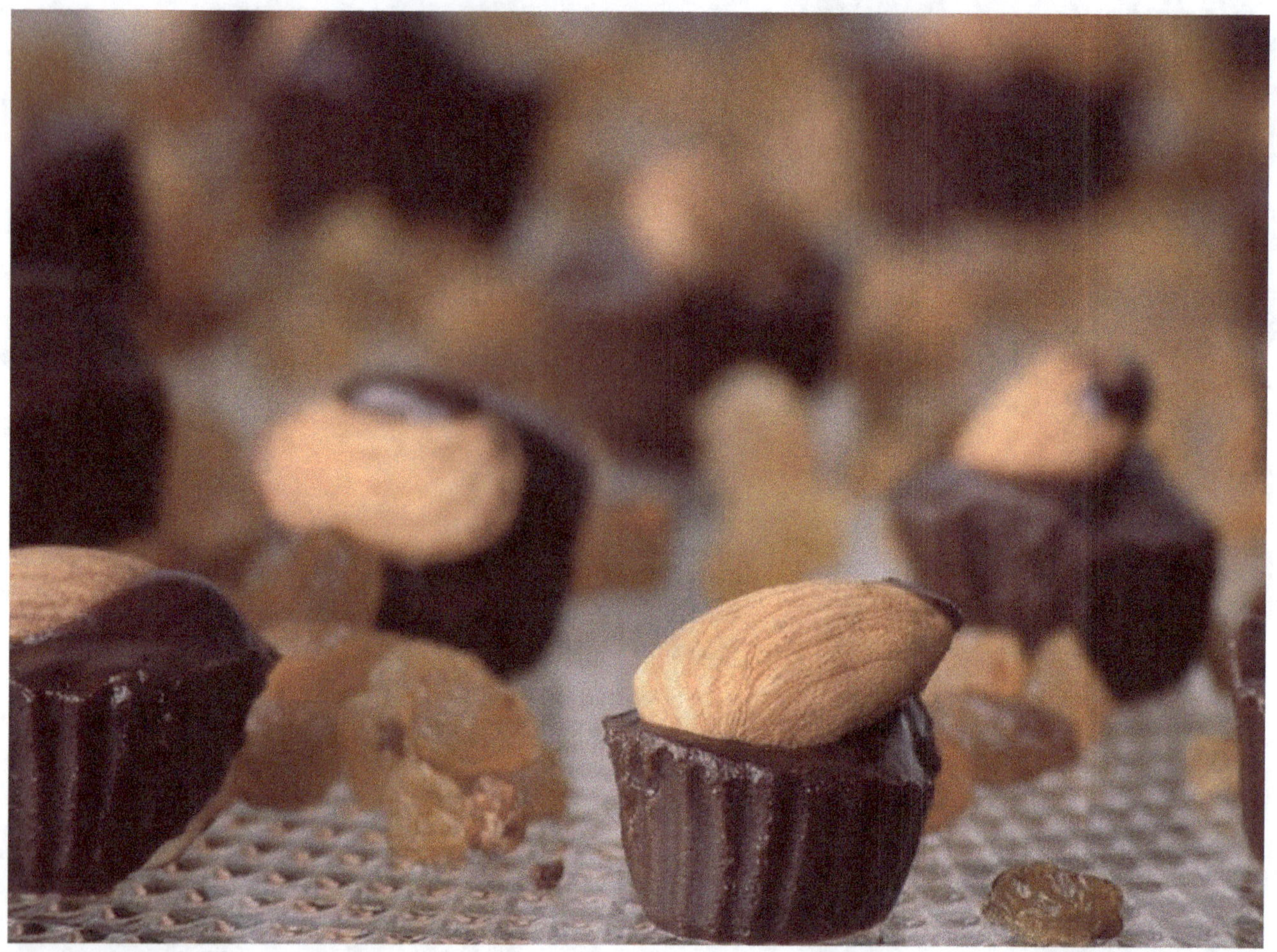

What You'll Need:

- 4 oz dark chocolate
- ¼ cup chopped almonds

Directions:

- Melt dark chocolate in a microwave or double boiler.
- Stir in chopped almonds.
- Spread mixture on a parchment-lined baking sheet.
- Chill until set, then break into pieces.

APPLE CRISP

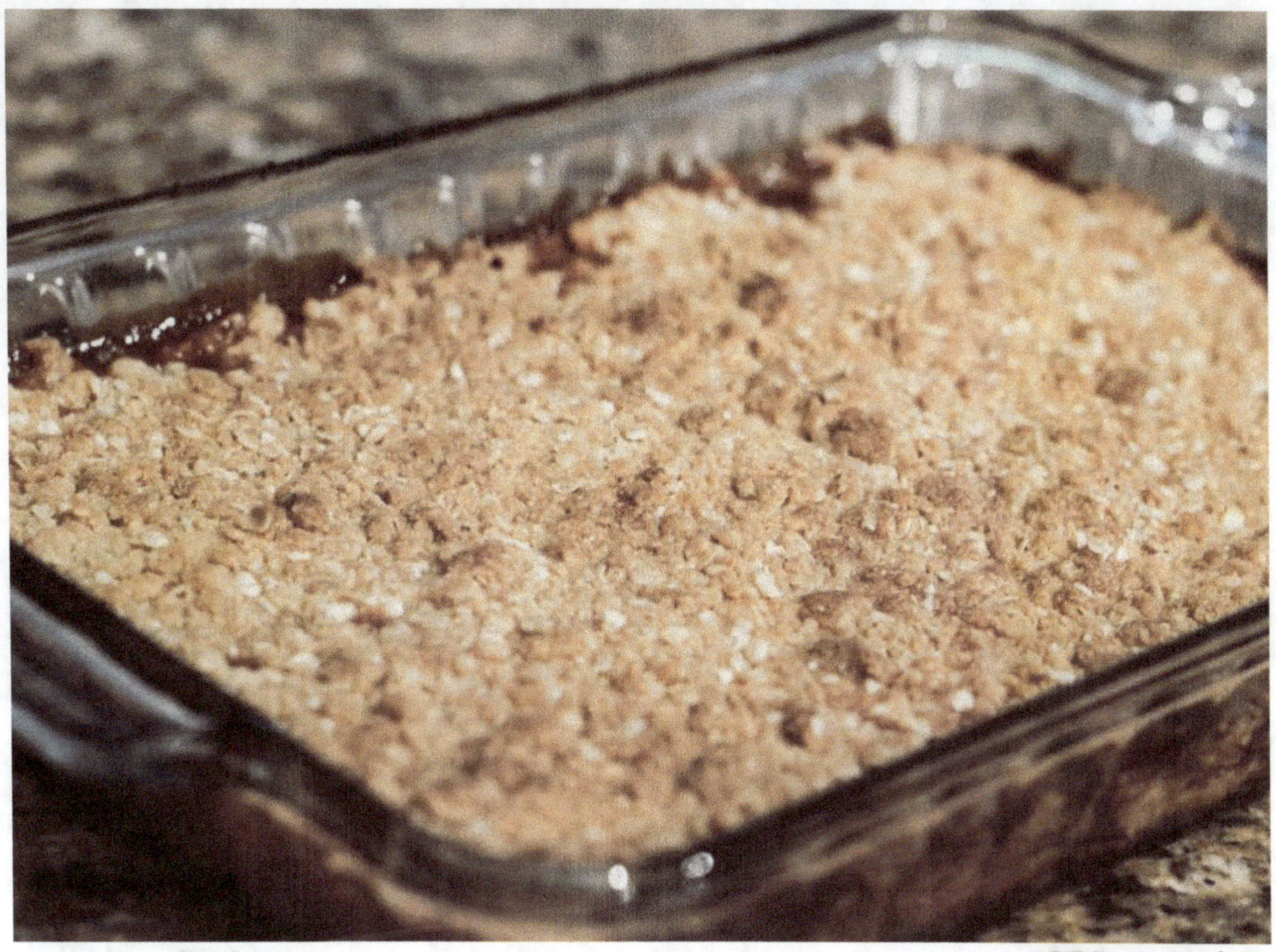

300 calories

<u>**What You'll Need:**</u>

- 3 apples, peeled and sliced
- ¼ cup oats
- ¼ cup brown sugar
- 2 tbsp butter
- 1 tsp cinnamon

<u>Directions:</u>

- Preheat oven to 350°F (175°C).
- Mix apples with cinnamon and place in a baking dish.
- Combine oats, brown sugar, and butter, then sprinkle over apples.
- Bake for 30–35 minutes until apples are tender.

BAKED PEARS WITH HONEY

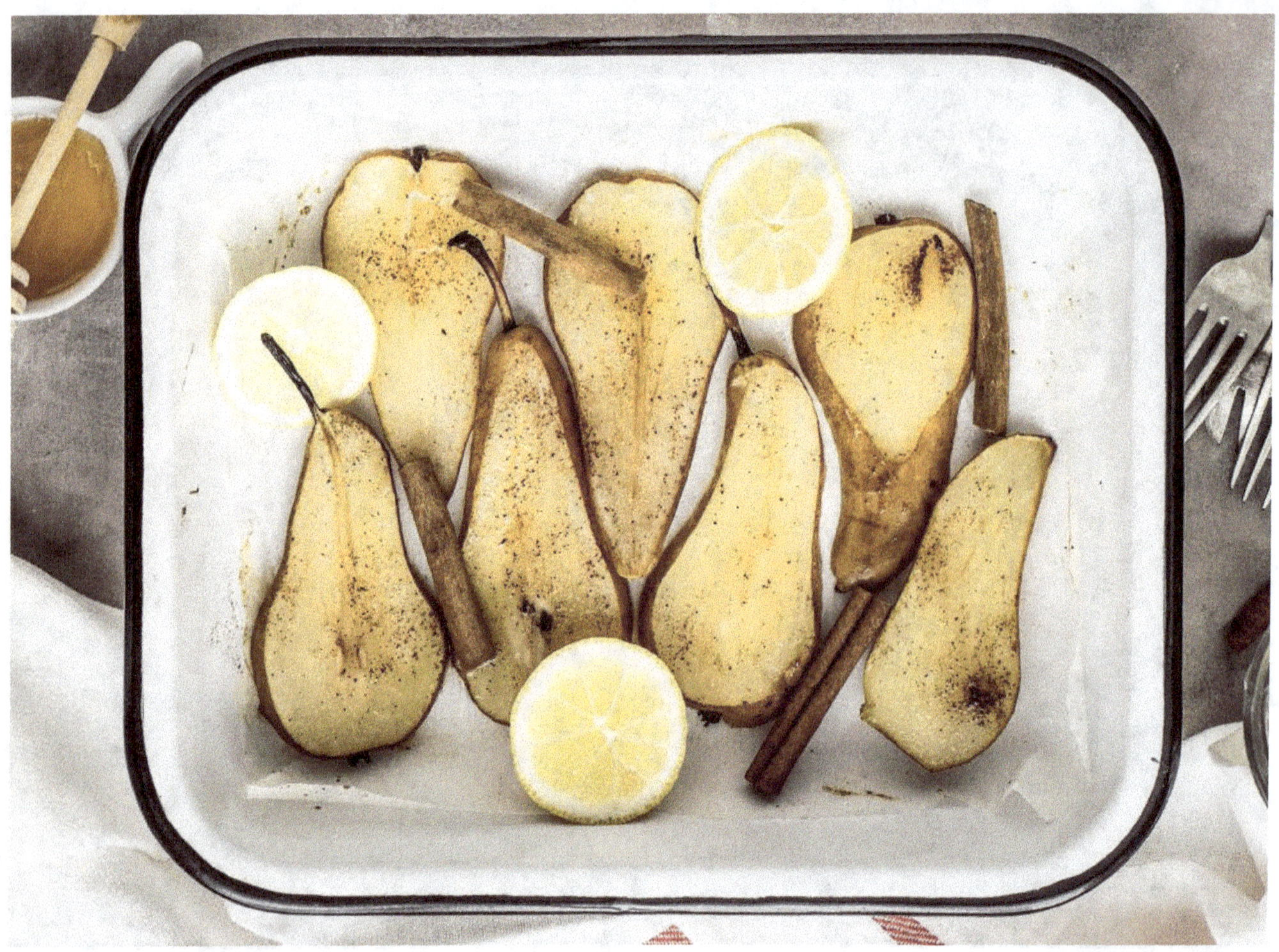

200 calories

What You'll Need:

- 2 pears, halved and cored
- 2 tbsp honey
- ½ tsp cinnamon

Directions:

- Preheat oven to 375°F (190°C).
- Place pears in a baking dish, drizzle with honey, and sprinkle with cinnamon.
- Bake for 20–25 minutes until tender.

FROZEN YOGURT

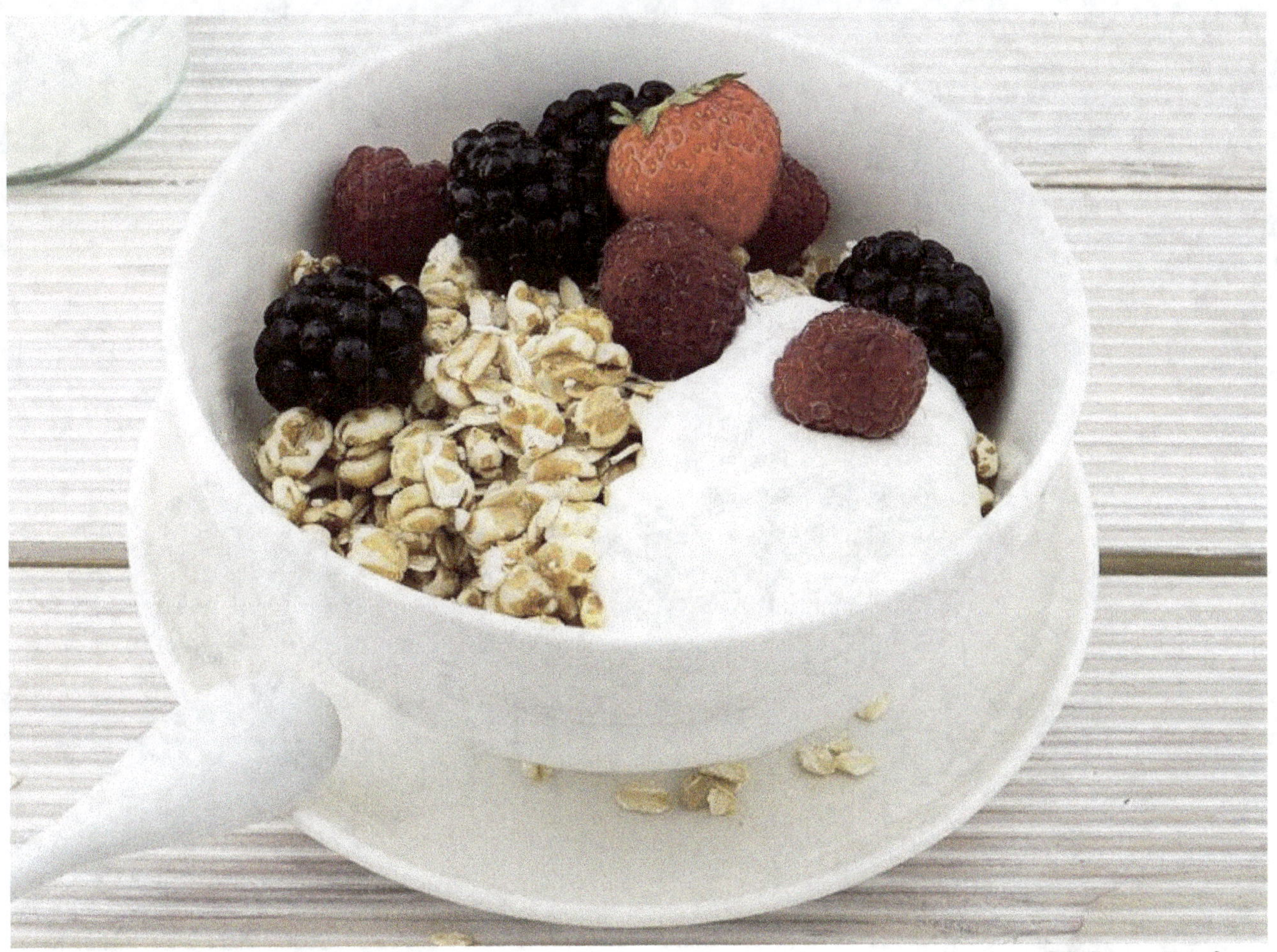

200 calories

What You'll Need:

- 1 cup Greek yogurt
- 2 tbsp honey
- ¼ cup mixed berries
- 2 tbsp granola

Directions:

- Mix Greek yogurt with honey and spread on a parchment-lined baking sheet.
- Top with mixed berries and granola.
- Freeze until firm, then break into pieces.

CHOCOLATE AVOCADO MOUSSE

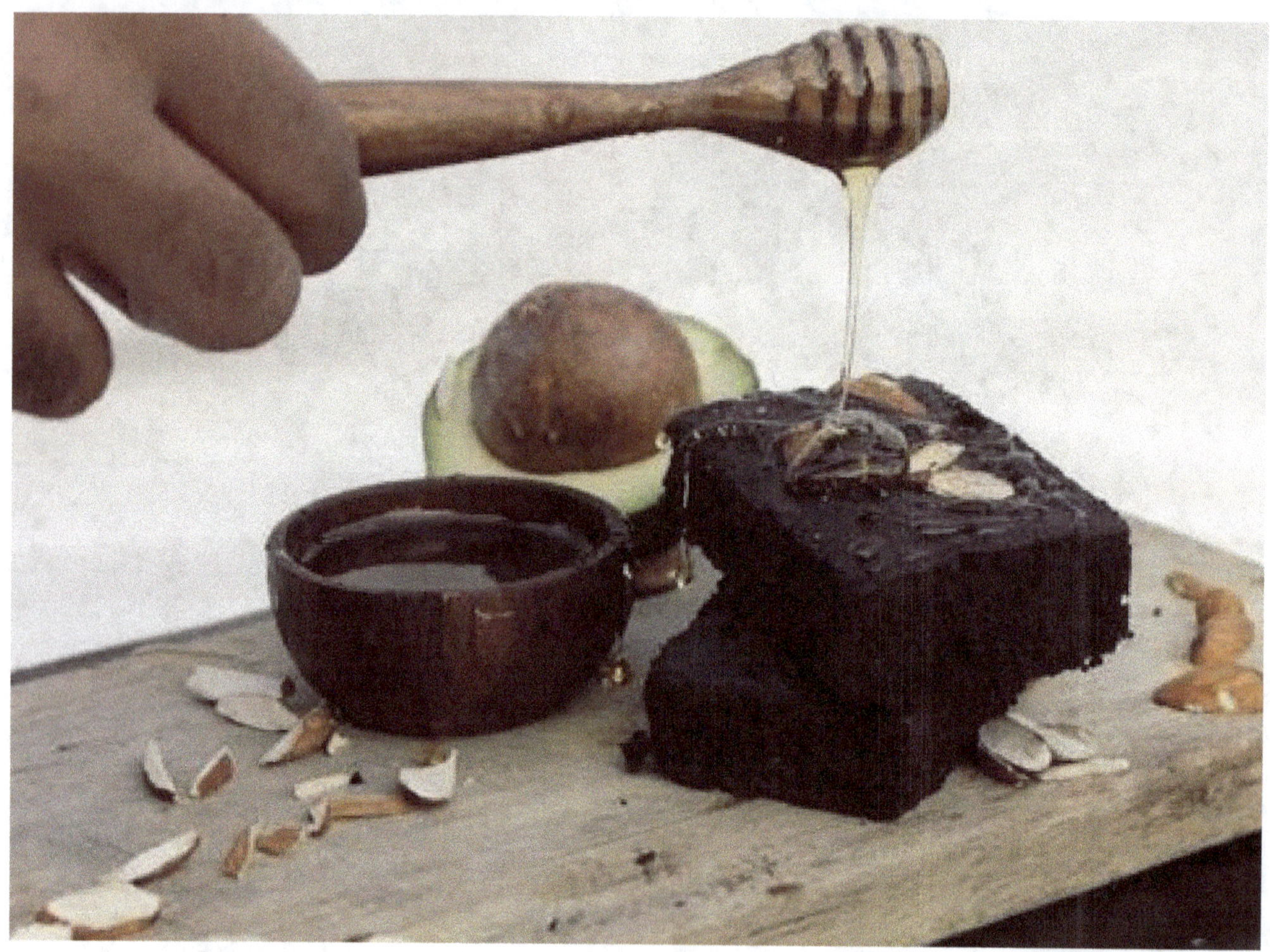

What You'll Need:

- 1 ripe avocado
- 2 tbsp cocoa powder
- 2 tbsp honey or maple syrup
- 1 tsp vanilla extract
- A pinch of salt

Directions:

- Scoop the avocado into a blender.
- Add cocoa powder, honey (or maple syrup), vanilla extract, and salt.
- Blend until smooth and creamy.
- Chill in the refrigerator for 30 minutes before serving.

BANANA OAT COOKIES

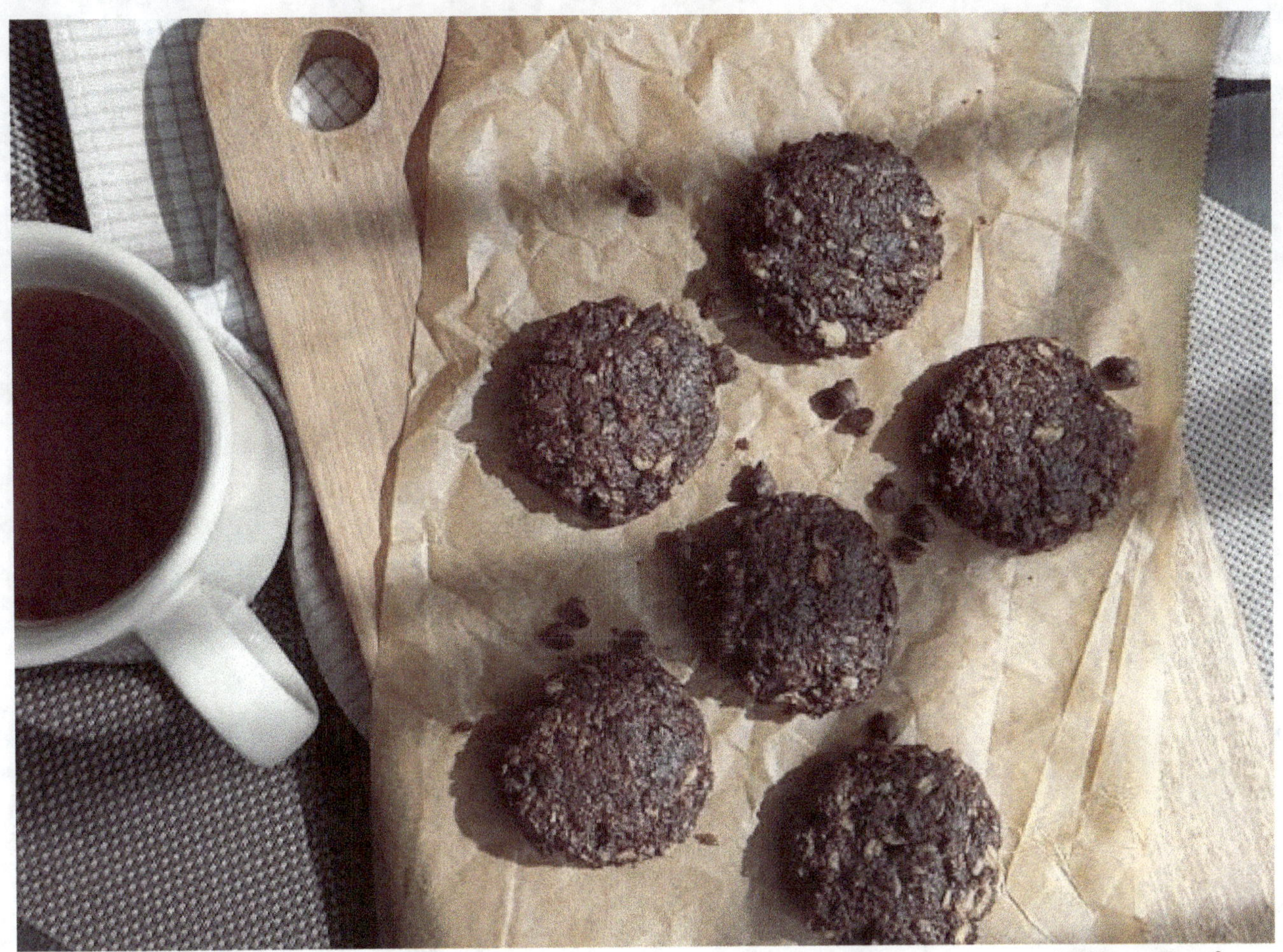

150 calories

What You'll Need:

- 2 ripe bananas, mashed
- 1 cup rolled oats
- 1/4 cup chocolate chips
- 1 tsp vanilla extract

Directions:

- Preheat the oven to 350°F (175°C).
- In a bowl, combine mashed bananas, rolled oats, chocolate chips, and vanilla extract.
- Drop a spoonful of the mixture onto a baking sheet lined with parchment paper.
- Bake for 12–15 minutes until the edges are golden brown.
- Let cool before serving.

www.ingramcontent.com/pod-product-compliance
Lightning Source LLC
Chambersburg PA
CBHW081309250726
48662CB00008B/2472